Healing the Dying

2ND EDITION

MELODIE OLSON
Ph.D., RN

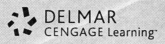

DELMAR
CENGAGE Learning™

Australia • Brazil • Japan • Korea • Mexico • Singapore • Spain • United Kingdom • United States

DELMAR
CENGAGE Learning™

**Healing the Dying,
Second Edition**
Melodie Olson

Health Care Publishing Director:
William Brottmiller

Product Development Manager:
Marion S. Waldman

Development Editor: Jill Rembetski

Editorial Assistant: Robin Irons

Executive Marketing Manager:
Dawn F. Gerrain

PTR Channel Manager: Gretta
Oliver

Production Editor: Mary Colleen
Liburdi

Cover Design: Mary Colleen Liburdi

For product information and technology assistance, contact us at
Cengage Learning Customer & Sales Support, 1-800-354-9706

For permission to use material from this text or product,
submit all requests online at **www.cengage.com/permissions**
Further permissions questions can be emailed to
permissionrequest@cengage.com

ISBN-13: 978-0-7668-2572-7

ISBN-10: 0-7668-2572-8

Delmar
Executive Woods
5 Maxwell Drive
Clifton Park, NY 12065
USA

Cengage Learning is a leading provider of customized learning solutions with office locations around the globe, including Singapore, the United Kingdom, Australia, Mexico, Brazil, and Japan. Locate your local office at **www.cengage.com/global**

Cengage Learning products are represented in Canada by Nelson Education, Ltd.

To learn more about Delmar, visit **www.cengage.com/delmar**

Purchase any of our products at your local bookstore or at our preferred online store **www.cengagebrain.com**

Notice to the Reader

Printed in the United States of America
6 7 8 9 10   16 15 14 13 12

FD031

For Larry

Contents

PART II   COMFORT OF THE DYING INDIVIDUAL

PART III   HELP FOR FAMILIES

PART IV   SPECIAL CASES

Preface

AIMS AND ORGANIZATION

Healing the Dying is intended to give the student and professional nurse practical guidance in the care of the dying patient, enabling the caregiver to improve the quality of care given. It is intended to update knowledge, and increase the range of choices for both the patient and the nurse so they can create an environment in which healing in its fullest sense can occur.

This second edition of *Healing the Dying* is organized similarly to the first edition; however, each chapter has been updated. We know much more about pain control than we did four years ago. We know more about how the physical body experiences shutting down, how to give spiritual assistance that is honestly helpful, and about legal issues that change over time. Cultural diversity and ethics are increasingly important in understanding how to care for the dying. All of these areas are expanded and timely in this edition.

Healing the Dying is organized into four parts. Part 1 includes epidemiology and theories related to dying. Grief theory, family theory, and other theories are helpful in understanding the kinds of care needed. Part 2 includes concepts of comfort for the individual. Measures to control discomfort, including sleep disturbance and mobility, are covered. Pain control, fear, and spiritual distress are also included. Part 3 focuses on family and social supports, such as hospice and bereavement services. Part 4 is a special section that considers relationships between particularly vulnerable populations of patients and nurses. The patients may have a common illness, such as cancer or HIV disease, or they may share some unique event, such as a near-death experience. They may be patients who are part of the nurse's family. Self-care hints for nurses are included (e.g., how to know when to take additional time off).

Vignettes are illustrations of themes that make the theories come alive. They are useful in making content clear and are included in every chapter.

The English language does not have a nonspecific gender pronoun. Rather than using the awkward he/she construction to avoid appearing sexist, people are referred to as he or she. An attempt is made to alternate gender-identifying pronouns when it is possible without causing confusion in the writing. Although nursing is still a predominantly female profession, men make substantial contributions to the nursing profession, as well as social work and all other patient-oriented caregiving professions, and are recognized in this book.

ACKNOWLEDGMENTS

Several people have encouraged the writing of this book, and this subsequent revision. As in the first edition, Lynne Keegan has been unfailingly supportive. It was she who had the vision to begin this incredibly useful series. The editors and staff of Delmar, Cengage Learning, especially Jill Rembetski, guided this revision so that the updates, pictures, and other timely additions that make it better, got done. Elaine Staller and Ramita Bonadonna contributed their skills and expertise in the first edition. In this changed and updated version, Nancee Sneed and Betsy Bateman Rothey contributed references, encouragement, and knowledge. Thank you all! I would also like to thank the following reviewers:

Joanne Bonicelli
Director of Complementary Therapy
Pikes Peak Hospice
Colorado Springs, CO 80903-5607

Lynn Keegan, RN, PhD, HNC, FAAN
Director Holistic Health Consultants
Port Angeles, Washington

John Nash
Social Worker/Bereavement Counselor
The Community Hospice
Albany, NY 12205

Ms. Cindy Petersen, BA
Hospice Program Manager
South Carolina Health and
    Human Services
Columbia, South Carolina

PART
I

The Sociology
of Death

CHAPTER 1

What Does it Mean to *Heal the Dying?*

DYING HEALED

Healing the dying sounds like an oxymoron, pulling together two contradictory thoughts. But to heal is not necessarily to cure, though that may happen during healing. To heal is to bring various levels of oneself—cellular, physical, intrapersonal, interpersonal, societal, spiritual, perhaps even cosmic—into new relationship with each other. Care of the person who is dying requires an assessment of the relationship of that person to self, others, and God, and appropriate intervention to assist with perceived deficits in these areas.

Dying *healed* means that a person has finished the business of life, said good-byes, and reached life's goals. An individual knows who he is and has a sense of integration of self and life. The dying person recognizes that this life was his own and no one else would have lived it the same way. His death matters to someone. Life's troubles have led to a kind of wisdom. Comfort and maybe even peace are achieved. The family has had sufficient time to grieve and to plan for the changes in the lives of its members. However, the time has not been excessive, leading to extreme emotional and physical fatigue and caregiver burnout. Control of the process of dying remains in the hands of the dying person for as long as he is able and willing to take it, fighting the good fight. When he is ready, decision making is passed to others, and a feeling of comfort results from their ministrations. Dying is perceived as a stage of life that fits into a broader philosophy giving both death and life meaning.

Dying *healed* is a process. Few people will achieve all of the goals inherent in the process. For some, there has not been time to grieve and to plan as one would wish. For some, caregiver burnout is a reality because of limited resources and very difficult expectations. For a few, physical comfort is difficult to achieve because of the disease process. In almost all cases, with knowledgeable care and support, a person who is dying and his family can be assisted along the process toward healing relationships, comfort, and peace in dying.

HEALING AS RELATIONSHIP

The notion of healing as relationship, different from curing, is an idea seen as early as Nightingale's work (1860/1969). She wrote that the role of the nurse was to put the patient in the best possible condition so that healing could occur. Nightingale believed that the physician removed impediments to healing with surgical techniques, medications, and other medical interventions. The nurse created the appropriate environment, which was clean, airy, and cheerful, and met the nutritional requirements of the individual. After that, it was the patient who did the work. Healing came from within each person.

Nightingale's most publicized patients were those soldiers injured during the Crimean War. Like veterans of all times, their scars were evidence of physical healing. The wounds were cleaned, foreign objects and bacteria removed, gangrenous or badly mangled limbs removed by amputation, and the wound edges brought together. Healing occurred through the body's own processes of clot formation, tissue regrowth, and the immune response. These are all internal processes. The cells came into new relationship with each other. Diseases were avoided or overcome.

Scars that give evidence of healing may disrupt other relationships. A livid scar on the face may interfere with self-esteem. Disruption of self-esteem may end a love affair. An amputated limb may disrupt a profession or affect one's economic status in life. An organ that was removed may interfere with one's stamina and limit activity. Perception of the scar, or changed relationships in one's physical body, can result in bitterness, loss of friends, loss of faith, loss of meaning.

Conversely, one can view the scar with thankfulness for the healing and begin to see past the scar. A person can begin to socialize with people for whom the scar is not a barrier. There is the possibility of achieving great satisfaction in life even with disability. Jim Abbott, born without a right hand, did not allow the lack of that hand to stop him from becoming a baseball pitcher for the Yankees. He pitched a no-hitter in the major leagues, a remarkable feat for anyone. In overcoming adversity, one develops abilities and a depth of meaning previously unknown. Friends are not limited by superficial artifacts. One learns new ways of interacting with family. A positive self-image strengthens.

Dying is a process that has many of the same characteristics as the process of scar formation. Both the scar and the dying processes cause physical change. The difference is that the scar is evidence of healing, while physical changes due to the disease process lead quite directly to the patient's death. For example, a cancerous growth may erode a necessary vascular route, causing bleeding. The skills needed to cope with the physical changes brought about by scarring or by dying are rooted in developing an awareness of the changes those processes require. Addressing those changes requires the willingness to establish and maintain a clear sense of self, and how the self relates to others.

Throughout the dying process, new relationships are forming. Perception of one's self as a dying individual could lead to loss of self-esteem, bitterness, loss of faith, loss of a sense of meaning in life. Perception of the dying person by others may also disrupt friendships and family relationships. But the dying process, like the scar, does not require that the changed relationships are negative, sad, or bitter. Persons who have been close to death but became well again often report that they have a new sense of living each moment more fully, of experiencing life with reverence, awe, and real joy. People who know they are dying sometimes capture that same spirit of satisfaction through integration of self. It is not that they want to die. A woman who was dying believed that several years prior to the current illness she had been given a new life. She had avoided death during a critical illness. Though now close to death with leukemia, she still hoped for another miracle—a postponement of death. During the first brush with death she feared the process of death. Would it hurt? What would physical symptoms be like? Is there anything that happens after the body stops breathing? None of these questions concerned her during the last stages of the leukemia. Instead, her reasons for wanting to stay a while longer on this earth were because her relationships with her grown children had become so precious she wanted to cherish them a while longer. This woman did not fear death, but lived in awe of each moment. She knew her children would be fine without her, but she had much joy in their presence. The first brush with death had gotten her beyond the fear, into a new sense of living each day fully. She sensed that when it was her time to die she would be willing to leave the family and let go of this life peacefully.

Mr. Bower

Mr. Bower was a 49-year-old veteran of the Korean War, who was hospitalized in a Veteran's Administration Hospital with cancer of the prostate. Because of his age, treatment was aggressive. Because he had very little support other than the Veteran's Administration, he was hospitalized for eight months before his death, with only a few weekend passes. During that time, he taught one young nurse about dying by sharing his experiences with her.

Ms. F. was a night nurse with two years of critical care experience. She had recently transferred to Mr. Bower's unit. About 3 A.M. of the second night she was there, Ms. F. found Mr. Bower smoking in the solarium. He wanted to talk. She sat with him for a few minutes, and began a pattern of relationship that lasted for the eight months they were both on the unit. Each night she was on duty, Mr. Bower waited up for her to talk more about dying. Some nights she was unable to find the time to talk, but on the nights that she did, Mr. Bower taught Ms. F. what it was like to face death and the many choices one has to make to continue to deepen the meaning of one's life. Mr. Bower was a person who died having achieved peace and purpose. He continues to share some of his lessons in this book.

Many people have ideas about what they want when they are dying. Often, people would like to be conscious very near the time of death, alert, and able to communicate. Dying in one's sleep is also acceptable, but not following a prolonged coma, or drawn out period of time. Most people do not want a period of suffering and/or pain, but if it is unavoidable, they would like to bear the burden with grace. People want to be treated with respect and dignity; they do not want to be abandoned by loved ones, professional people, or society. Most people recognize that there is no guarantee of a peaceful death, so they may need to grow in courage (Callahan, 1993; Webb, 1997).

PALLIATIVE CARE AND HEALING

Healing the dying requires attention to relationship. In caring for the dying patient, the caregiver understands that the medical prognosis of the patient is limited and care is termed *palliative*. Care focuses on quality of life rather than length of life. The World Health Organization defines palliative care as:

> The active total care of patients whose disease is not responsive to curative treatment. Control of pain, of other symptoms and of psychological, social, and spiritual problems, is paramount. The goal of palliative care is achievement of the best quality of life for patients and their families.

They add:

> Palliative care . . . affirms life and regards dying as a normal process . . . neither hastens nor postpones death, . . . provides relief from pain and other distressing symptoms, . . . integrates the psychological and spiritual aspects of care, . . . offers a support system to help patients live as actively as possible until death, . . . offers a support system to help families cope during the patient's illness and their own bereavement (Doyle, Hanks, & McDonald, 1993; World Health Organization, 1990).

The concept of healing the dying incorporates palliative care and goes beyond to nurture relationships of all kinds, to provide choices so that the dying patient can create an environment in which life can be lived to its fullest, and at some point, the patient can make the choice to let go and slip into a peaceful death. The nurse or other health care provider is in full and healthy partnership with the patient during this time.

Palliative care requires certain abilities, and many of them are defined as relationship. Of the 15 care competencies identified by the American Association of Colleges of Nursing (1998) necessary for nurses to provide high quality care to the dying and their families, skills that reflect the ability to establish, maintain, or support relationships are included in at least six. Examples include effective and compassionate communication; demonstration of respect for other's attitudes, feelings, values, and expectations; collaboration with an interdisciplinary team; assisting patient, family, colleagues, and self with grief and suffering. Ferrell (1999) suggests that good end of life care is that care we would seek for ourselves or our loved ones if faced with a terminal illness. That care includes palliation; symptom management (sometimes aggressively); good communication of prognosis and options for treatment; policy, ethics, and legal issues involving drug restrictions; and advanced directives and bereavement services. Care competencies support a "good death," identified by Steinhauser (2000) as having "pain and symptom management, clear decision making, preparation for death, completion, contributing to others, and affirmation of the whole person."

Recognizing that the nurse will always feel some emotion when a patient dies opens the nurse to sharing the experience rather than denying it, dealing with often contradictory emotions. The nurse is in the environment of the dying patient, and contributes to that milieu. Making choices about care that allow the patient to live according to his wishes while following established standards of care, and caring for other patients at the same time, requires skill, knowledge, compassion, organization, and a willingness to confront one's own mortality. One way to begin the process of being able to confront one's own mortality is to consciously and intentionally plan one's own death. Anyone who chooses a profession that involves caring for the dying will learn from the exercise of planning an ideal death. Ask yourself some of the following questions:

1. What would an ideal death be like?

2. Would you like to be alone or with friends and family when you die? If not alone, with whom?

3. What would you like to tell those you love before you die?

4. Are there issues in your life that require you to forgive or to ask forgiveness?

5. What rituals would you like for the period after your death (e.g., memorial service, cremation, funeral)? What kind of ceremony, if any?

6. Have you taken care of legal issues, such as advanced directives, a will, and care for pets?

7. What have been the most precious events in your life? (Olson & Dossey, 2000)

Many of the same issues the patient confronts in his dying are issues the nurse confronts in helping that person to live in the time allotted—issues of physical, spiritual, and psychological distress, and the need for support of different kinds. Caring for the dying patient requires caring for one's self.

SUMMARY

Healing includes new relationships between all levels of the person, leading to a feeling of well-being, safety, and peace. Healing leads to greater comfort. Healing the dying helps the dying person to a perception of life as having been meaningful. Healing the dying may occur in the presence of disease if the death ultimately is peaceful.

REFERENCES

American Association of Colleges of Nursing (1998). Peaceful Death. Presentation at the meeting of Robert Wood Johnson End-of-Life Roundtable, November 11–12, 1997, Washington D.C.

Callahan, D. (1993, July–August). *Pursuing a peaceful death* (pp. 33–38). Hasting's Center Report.

Doyle, D., Hanks, G. W. C., & MacDonald, N. (Eds.). (1993). *Oxford textbook of palliative medicine*. Oxford: Oxford University Press.

Ferrell, B. (1999). Caring at the end of life. *Reflections, 31–37.*

Nightingale, F. (1969). *Notes on nursing*. New York: Dover. (Original work published 1860)

Olson, M., & Dossey, B. M. (2000). Dying in peace. In Dossey, B. M., Keegan, L., & Guzzetta, C. E. (Eds.), *Holistic nursing: A handbook for practice* (pp. 661–684). Gaithersburg, MD: Aspen Publications.

Steinhauser, K. E., Clipper, E. C., McNeilly, M., Christakis, N. A., McIntyre, L. M., & Tulsky, J. A. (2000). In search of a good death: Observations of patients, families and providers. *Annals of Internal Medicine, 132* (10), p. 825–832.

Webb, M. (1997). *The good death*. New York: Bantam Books.

World Health Organization. (1990). *Cancer pain relief and palliative care* (Technical Report Series 804). Geneva: Author.

The Sociology of
Patterns and Values

THE RELATIONSHIP OF DEATH AND SOCIETY

Societal values determine attitudes and behaviors related to death and healing. How an individual feels about death and what actions are taken as a response to those feelings are based in part on what society values as appropriate behavior. It is important to identify society's values because contemporary American society relies on those values when addressing death-related social issues, and how people should behave. Those issues include extending life with technology past the time people would wish, euthanasia, abortion, capital punishment, the nature of a peaceful death, and other death-related social events. Knowing society's values helps people begin to create an environment in which each person can die peacefully. One way to begin to identify society's values in relation to death is to examine language, symbols, and rituals of death in any culture.

Language and Symbols

Language is the set of symbols by which people communicate, and how they identify what is important and meaningful in life. A society that values esthetics highly will have a language rich in imagery and vivid description. A society that values scientific thought will have precise definitions of events and be concise, almost terse, by comparison to the more descriptive speech. Describing the passage of blood through the heart in some New Guinea languages takes a whole morning, as each part of each

...mber is described in detail. In English, only a few sentences are necessary to list the structures passed and their functions as blood travels the short route. The use of a short, specific vocabulary for science illustrates the value the scientist places on efficiency and clarity of thought. The simpler the sentence, the more useful the concept.

The number of words a culture has for a subject, reflecting its many meanings, may be a clue to the importance of that subject for the people, and how they deal with it. In many languages, there are several words for the concept of love. Those words reflect a love of parents for children, a physical relationship with another adult, a love for God. The willingness of people to use those words and discuss the subject reflects in part how comfortable they are with the topic. A lack of words for a concept may mean that the people do not think in terms of that concept. Few words for a subject or the use of euphemism in place of those words may indicate a denial of the reality of the concept.

For some people in the United States, death is a difficult word to use. The difficulty in telling someone that he or she is dying, to discuss the impending death with family and others, or to say someone is dead at the time of the funeral reflects attitudes of the group toward death. Death becomes more tolerable if the dying one is lost, or goes to her eternal rest. Such language suggests a societal denial of death, a collusion to avoid the pain that death brings. Even death by violence may sound almost acceptable if, instead of killing someone, you waste or terminate the enemy, or put someone to sleep. It is also possible to sensitize the population to death by linking the word with other words, thus softening its meaning, as in death by chocolate, dead ahead, or you're dead right.

The language used by people not only reflects values, but changes their values in relation to the topic. Euphemisms people use are the first experiences the next generation has with the idea. Children learn that the player with the football is dead meat before they learn how it feels to miss Grandma when she dies. Society as a whole may sanction or withhold sanction for actions involving death depending on how the topic is addressed. For example, a physician may talk of *euthanasia,* a technical term, while a writer of novels terms the act a *mercy killing.* As euthanasia becomes linked with mercy, laws are more likely to change, and society seeks to find ways in which to implement the basic value of mercy.

Healing, too, reflects societal attitudes. Common usage of the term may imply religious belief to those who attend and participate in healing services at their local places of worship. The term may reflect a precise physiological pattern, as in wound healing. It is often taken to mean cure of disease, or it may mean resolution of some problem. Generally, healing is positive. Things people do to achieve healing are accepted, even when they take place outside of the common plan of action or usually approved activities, so long as they do not harm others. For example, megavitamin therapies have not been shown to be efficacious in traditional studies, but cancer patients who are dying are not prohibited from taking them if they go to herb shops or nutrition centers. Doctors generally do not prescribe the vitamins because they are not within accepted standards of medical practice.

Healing is often adopted as a positive philosophy when a society is dissatisfied with the medical care of the times. There were several periods of holistic health movements in the United States during which vitamin therapy, special baths, herbs, and other nutrients were popularized and given status as adjuncts or aids to healing (Hamilton, 1991). Various healers such as curanderos, shamans, and religious leaders were given high status, followed or at least heard. They commonly espoused a path to a positive life—not necessarily disease free, but healthy as a whole. Almost always, interpersonal relationships were stressed by these healers.

Art

Another set of symbols that society uses to express its values and attitudes toward death and healing is art in its many forms. A life-size mural on a wall in an inner city neighborhood depicting a knife dripping blood suspended above the body of a teenager focuses attention on violence and societal tensions. The same sized mural depicting the death of Christ painted on the wall of a church focuses on religious meanings of death. A Diego Rivera larger-than-life mural on the walls of government buildings in Mexico City makes a political statement about death. These social, religious, or political statements may contribute to an understanding of the many meanings of death.

Similarly, music that focuses on death may create a sense of sadness, as in "Ode to Billy Joe," where death occurred in youth and by choice; or as in the traditional dirge music played at the funerals of many former U.S. presidents. Music may also uplift spirits, as in traditional religious music pieces like Handel's *Messiah.* It ends with a joyous celebration of immortality—the belief that at least spiritually, there is no death.

Drama, literature, and other forms of art also reflect and change societal attitudes toward death and healing (see Figure 2-1). The intense emotion of a man confronting his own mortality in Ingmar Bergman's classic film *Wild Strawberries* has haunted a generation. The need for healing of Willie Loman, in *Death of a Salesman,* shouts to the audience. Current ethical debate about the effect of watching violent death daily on television, and its potential contribution to increasing rates of acts of violence, is evidence of the power of the media in influencing attitudes and behaviors.

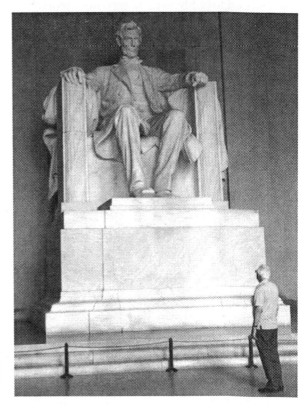

Figure 2-1
The Lincoln Memorial is a work of art that creates a feeling of awe without using words.

Ritual

One reason that art in its many forms is so powerful is that it often makes use of the rituals of death. Rituals of death include:

- *people,* including funeral directors, nurses and physicians, clergy, and others who are associated with the dying

- *places,* such as cemeteries, battlefields, and funeral chapels, which exist either to honor the dead or to provide a special place for rites to occur

- *special times* for remembrance of the dead, such as Veteran's Day or Memorial Day

- *special objects* associated with death, such as obituaries, hearses, and tombstones

- *special symbols,* such as skull and crossbones or a black arm band (Doyle, Hanks, & MacDonald, 1993, p. 34)

Melding these symbols of death and dying can provide a rich tapestry for art, connected with both rational study and emotion, and rooted in the values of the people—the things they consider right or wrong. The images they portray become the patterns of behavior that are followed in life as people come to believe this is the correct way to behave. One comes to believe that suicide is wrong when a powerful poem conveys the suffering of parents following the suicide death of a teen. Although desensitization to suicide may occur if the word or concept is simply repeated in a superficial way many times, desensitization does not seem to occur when art gives the term feeling and connection to self, when it becomes personal.

Rituals of death are also rooted in the culture. Cultures may view death in several ways. Some cultures are death-accepting, and others are death-denying. Some may even be termed death-defying (Kearl, 1989, p. 26). Death may be a process, or a state. Cultures may view death as an end to life, or as a transition to another form of life. If it is seen as a transition, the concept of immortality may be one of personal transition or of collective transition. Hindus believe that the life between reincarnations is the real (or objective) world, and that the current life is an illusion. Americans, on the other hand, generally believe what is felt, seen, and heard is real, and the notion of another world is quite illusory. Even so, the illusory world past death holds promise for another kind of life, and so funeral customs may be as much a passage to another life as a farewell to this one.

Historically, funeral and burial rites have been both symbolic and useful. They reinforce beliefs of a society about death. For example, the kings of Egypt, buried as Tutankhamen was, with food, riches, personal keepsakes, and treasures, reinforced the belief of the time that such items would be of value in the hereafter. That contrasts with modern views of Americans who believe that "you can't take it with you." An expensive coffin in the United States is more often a sign of respect for the dead than an attempt to influence what happens after burial.

Funeral rites are comforting to individuals as they realize they are part of a greater whole, a family or a clan (see Figure 2-2). Rites provide a place to begin the bereavement process, to talk safely and without the discomfort that so often accompanies conversation about death, especially in a death-denying society. Jews traditionally cover mirrors and light special candles when they sit Shiva. The rites often include a

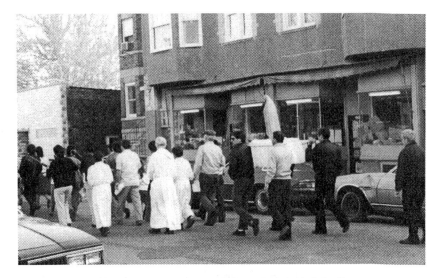

Figure 2-2 Funeral processions are rituals that help families and communities deal with the loss of a loved one.

wake—a visitation with family and friends for mutual support and comfort. At a traditional Irish wake, family and friends remember, toast, and celebrate the deceased. Sometimes the rites provide a place and a formal time to say good-bye to the person who has died or to complete unfinished business with that person. An adult child, called home after the death of a parent, may look at the familiar face in the coffin and kiss it one last time, or say "thank you" for the things not recognized before, or just say "good-bye." To remember one who has been cremated, the ashes may be scattered in a place of personal meaning, leading to a release of grief. Rites are society's way of creating a structure in which a set of behaviors is taught to help members of that society deal with grief and loss, or to celebrate and memorialize group members. That structure changes slowly over time as societal values and attitudes change.

MORTALITY THROUGH THE AGES

Mr. Bower, whom we met in Chapter 1, lived in the hospital with his disease for eight months. He could do so because of the technology and care available to treat him. He was 49 years old when he died. That is approximately the number of years he could have been expected to live if he had been born in England in 1900 (Lancaster, 1990, p. 44). For most citizens of the United States, 49 years seems young. In fact, in 1989, the life expectancy for white men born in the United States was 73 years (U.S. Bureau of the Census, 1992). A man who was 73 years old in 1989 would have lived through several periods of high mortality rates (his first year of life; his teenage years, prone to infection and/or violence; middle-age years, which predisposed him to cardiovascular disease and some cancers). Having survived those things, he could be expected to live another 10 years.

Minority groups have a somewhat shorter life expectancy than the cultural majority groups. This is most likely related to the greater proportion of minority groups living in restricted economic conditions. Inner city violence kills more minority teens than Caucasian teens, sometimes because of gang culture, and often because they happen to live in a certain area in which violence is endemic. Some diseases such as diabetes and cardiovascular disease are more deadly in groups with limited access to health care. That limited access may be due to distance from a health care setting, insufficient numbers of health care professionals in an area, or too few resources with which to purchase care. Diseases specific to cultural groups, such as Thalassemia, or diseases that affect only a few people, such as multiple sclerosis, may receive fewer research dollars, so cure may be delayed. Diseases that affect a minority group of people may require expensive treatments that few people can afford. The only known possible cure for sickle cell anemia, a disease affecting primarily African American people, is bone marrow transplant. That treatment is not only extremely expensive, but depends on finding appropriate bone marrow donors. Although matches between donors and those needing bone marrow will be found most frequently in a similar racial group (because blood types are genetically determined), African Americans have a low rate of giving blood or organs for transplant. If this trend continues for bone marrow, the cure for sickle cell anemia will not be widely available.

Mortality Before the Industrial Revolution

How long a person is likely to live, and how she is likely to die, is largely a function of the society and the times in which she lives. Before the industrial revolution, a typical deathbed scene involved a young mother and father desperately trying to save the feverish infant who was so young its only means of expression was to cry. Too often, the parents were unsuccessful. Nearly as likely was the deathbed scene in which the mother, having had several children already, died during childbirth. The youthful widower was left with the other children, sometimes a newborn, and often without the means to care for them all. The newborn may have died of starvation if a wet nurse could not be found because lack of refrigeration prevented storing milk.

Mortality rates for any one region varied according to the presence or absence of epidemic, for which there was no known cure, or of famine, an equally uncontrollable event. Contagious diseases afflicted those who lived along popular highways or in dense populations, and those who had little resistance to disease. Contributing to inadequate resistance to disease was poor nutritional status, almost nonexistent hygiene (lack of running water, sewer systems), and other environmental factors.

From the Industrial Revolution to World War II

After the industrial revolution, social conditions began to change. Working conditions improved, and there were developments in agriculture, housing, sanitation, communication, and public health. People born in 1930 had a life expectancy of over 60 years. By the 1950s, life expectancy in the United States was over 70 years. With a few exceptions, most notably the development of antibiotics and widespread use of vaccines, medical developments were not credited for the extension of life expectancy. Social change was believed responsible for increasing the number of years of life. Social change is in the hands of the public, and the changes created were based on the values of the times.

Deathbed scenes after the industrial revolution moved to the older aged groups. People died at home during the first part of the twentieth century, more often of prolonged disease, such as cancer, and of infections such as tuberculosis or meningitis. They had time to call in the family to the bedside, and name their heirs, say good-bye, and give their blessings to the caregivers and loved ones. In the second half of the twentieth century, two major shifts occurred that changed the way people thought of and dealt with death.

Post World War II

During World War II, the role of women began changing rapidly. Women worked in industry during the war, and did not give up their jobs after the war. Immediately after the war, many families became dependent on the incomes of two adults or a single head of household when there was only one adult in the home. Fewer women took on the traditional role of full-time housewife and family caretaker. When family members, particularly the aged, became ill, they were hospitalized, often for extended periods of time. Eventually, it became the norm for the person who was not going to get well to complete the dying process in the hospital, though all the hospital staff could accomplish was palliative care. By tacit agreement, hospitalization was prolonged, in part so that the family could continue with their work without interruption. Their paid sick days covered only the employee, so lost days of work meant lost pay at the time when money was needed to cover the expenses of the sick or dying family member. The longer the hospital was willing to keep the patient (covered by insurance, of course), the fewer days off the caregiver had to take. Society had not defined the appropriate place or caregiver of palliative care. Hospice was valued, but not yet widespread. Home care was viewed as difficult, and people unskilled in caregiving did not know what their roles were. In the early part of the century, private duty nurses were available and were hired by the wealthy to care for loved ones at home until they died. In the decades between 1950 and 1990, the most common model of care took place in the hospital, given or supervised by professional nurses.

The advent of prospective payment system (payment for hospitalization based on diagnosis and the average length of time a person needed hospital care for reasons related to medical and nursing care) ended the use of hospitals for extended maintenance care. But a whole generation had grown up never seeing death, except in the special death place of the funeral home. Death occurred in hospitals, out of sight.

A second reason for the change in the way people thought of death in the second half of the twentieth century was the extended and seemingly ever increasing use of technology. The Korean and Vietnam wars are often credited with the initial explosion of the use of impressive technologic developments for trauma patients. Machines were developed to take over major functions of the body, like breathing (ventilators), exchanging body waste (dialysis), or monitoring functions such as electrical impulses (electroencephalography, cardiac telemetry), or pressures (ventricular screws or Swanz-ganz catheters). Nurses, physicians, and family members often felt caught in a kind of moral dilemma. The values of the American society as a whole suggested that all human life was worth preserving, that death was to be postponed, and that there was always the chance of the miracle in which the patient would suddenly become alert and whole. The cost in terms of dignity of the patient, possible pain, and other kinds of suffering was overridden by the finality of death and the implication that everything possible was not done for the person. Family members would feel guilty if they considered financial ruin a cause for ending treatment, and health care team members felt a sense of failure when death occurred. Death deformed life; it was not a natural process.

Being present for the death of a loved one or having the dying person in the home, and believing that death should be avoided at all costs for as long as possible seems to have led many Americans to imagine a kind of *technologic death* because they have not seen a peaceful death. A technologic death occurs when a dying person is kept alive via a variety of machines. Many people have a vision of tubes in every opening of the body dripping fluid either in or out, sensors sending information translated into beeps, the soft bubbling and whoosh of artificial breathing, and personhood suspended in some unknown state. Although this view of death is often inaccurate, it is perpetuated by television and movies, often a worst case scenario. The process of death is feared, ironically, for the very lack of dignity that the available technology requires when used to prolong the end of life.

Some people would like to fight death to the end, and use every available resource to assist in the fight. They want to taste every drop of life, good or bad. Others wish to avoid the extremes and make choices based on other values, such as comfort or dignity. Legal issues regarding who has the right or the obligation to limit the use of technology to sustain life or prolong death and under what circumstances must be defined. Attempts to end the use of technology that is sustaining life can result in long delays and conflict between individuals, families, and society as represented by the law.

The legal problems encountered by people who want to limit the use of technology to extend life came about initially because of mandates intended to preserve and protect the public. Society feared that someone other than the dying individual would make an irrevocable decision to forgo life support contrary to the wishes of the person. Living wills and informed consent laws are society's attempts to give some choice about the dying process to those experiencing it. Without such choice, the modern deathbed scene usually takes place in the hospital, with the one who is dying surrounded by machines that make jarring noises and lights, and strangers who are busy with many tasks, who feel their responsibility is to fight death to the end. The wish for a peaceful death is a vague hope.

Death at Present

Without trauma due to accident or violence, people born in the United States have an even chance of living to the age of 85. Riley (1989, p. 11) called this the maximum average life span, or *modal age of death*. Some groups are at higher risk for earlier death, but researchers now agree that people probably have genetic limitations on life span, and that further prolongation of life without genetic change is unlikely. Others believe that the modal age of death will increase to a maximum achievable age of 110 in groups who make social changes toward maximum health. Even so, in the next decade the majority of deaths will occur either as technologic deaths in modern trauma centers, the result of increasing violence, suicide, and accident rates, or in old age. As political forces wrestle with health care reform issues, sites of extended care for the elderly are likely to be varied according to the social and economic status of the population. Some groups will value home care and learn the skills to care for the loved one who is dying. They will receive support from the larger society, and allow the elderly to die at home. Others will be comfortable receiving help from long-term care facilities. Family members will seek places where around-the-clock care will be provided in safe and pleasant surroundings, protecting the patient's choices and dignity. Those who wish to be present at the patient's death will be called, and new rituals will be created to meet the needs of the bereaved and the dying person. Callahan (1993) suggested that if society begins to value the idea of a peaceful death, everything that interferes with peace must be justified. This means that lights, tubes, noises, and people in the patient's environment would be limited to those that contribute to comfort. Doctors would have the responsibility of deciding when medical treatment would not serve to contribute to either cure or comfort. For example, if cardio-pulmonary resuscitation (CPR) were unlikely to be successful, it would not be started because to do so would only be an act of violence toward the dying patient (Youngner, 1988). Fighting for life at any cost would be seen as one choice of several. A peaceful death would become more common, more possible.

Political, economic, and ethical debates take place before society changes, and it is in those debates that nurses have the chance to influence how dying will occur for patients in the future. The debate takes place at all levels of society: in Congress during health care reform and in financing decisions; in think tanks like the Hastings Center for Ethics; in grassroots organizations; and in the institutions devoted to education, religion, and health care. For example, the Project on Death in America convened experts from a number of health care disciplines to develop a consensus and common understanding of core principles for end-of-life care (see Table 2-1). Many professional organizations have adopted the principles and are now working to eliminate legal and regulatory barriers to implementing them. These are all social institutions, and the nurse who wishes to remain informed about healing the dying needs to monitor and perhaps contribute to the debate.

TABLE 2-1	Core Principles for End-of-Life Care

Clinical policy at the end of life and the professional practice it guides should:

1. Respect the dignity of both patient and caregivers;
2. Be sensitive to and respectful of the patient's and family's wishes;
3. Use the most appropriate measures that are consistent with the patient choices;
4. Encompass alleviation of pain and other physical symptoms;
5. Assess and manage psychological, social, and spiritual/religious problems;
6. Offer continuity (the patient should be able to continue to be cared for, if so desired, by his/her primary care and specialist providers);
7. Provide access to any therapy which may realistically be expected to improve the patient's quality of life including alternative or nontraditional treatment;
8. Provide access to palliative care and hospice care;
9. Respect the right to refuse treatment;
10. Respect the physician's professional responsibility to discontinue some treatments when appropriate, with consideration for both patient and family preferences;
11. Promote clinical and evidence-based research on providing care at the end of life.

Cassel, C. K., & Foley, K. M. (1998). *Principles for care of patients at the end of life: An emerging consensus among the specialties of medicine.* New York: The Millbank Memorial Fund.

PEACEFUL DEATH: LETTING GO

Euthanasia, suicide, and prolonged extension of life past one's desire to live would not be issues today if people believed that they had the skill to decide to die, and then did so. There would be no need to consider some of the most important ethical issues of our time. But there is abundant evidence that people do have such abilities. It is well-documented that in many societies individuals die without a demonstrable physical cause. Sometimes it may be related to a sadness, as with Mr. Kashu. Sometimes the physical cause can be inferred, as in the case of Eskimo elders who, in the past, chose not to be a burden on their social group by floating away from the group on an ice floe when they felt that they had outlived their usefulness. One can imagine hypothermia, drowning, or starvation to be the cause of death. Sometimes the fact that a person believes that she will die seems sufficient to bring the death about.

Many cultures have a powerful spiritual person, shaman, or witch who has the ability to hex or cast a spell on a person, which causes sick-

Mr. Kashu

Mr. Kashu was planning to go home tomorrow. His pneumonia was almost resolved, as was seen on the chest x-ray. The antibiotics had been changed from I.V. to oral, so that he could take them at home and continue his recovery. On this day, the mail contained a letter from his married son, which he thought contained arrangements for going home. He was wrong. The short letter told him of his son's plan to divorce his wife. The son informed Mr. Kashu that the responsibility for the divorce was Mr. Kashu's because he had not helped his son enough over the years. The son blamed the father for everything that had gone wrong in his life. After reading the letter, the middle-aged man looked up and said, "It's time to die now." He lay on his bed and let go of his life. He was pronounced dead 30 minutes later. No physical cause could be found for his death.

ness or death without obvious physical contact. Voodoo priestesses in New Orleans were at one time thought to mix a variety of things, including the plaster from a broken statue of a saint and dirt from a fresh grave taken at midnight, and use the resulting powder to cause harm or death to enemies.

Conversely, most nurses and physicians know a patient who came to the hospital with a severe disease and was not expected to live. Yet years later the former patient is clearly a survivor, and no one knows why; many people with far fewer symptoms and less severe disease have died. It would seem that such people possess the quality of hardiness. They have the ability to hold onto life despite many challenges. Health care providers also know people who have lived long enough to achieve a goal in spite of great odds. Sometimes they live long enough to participate in some family event, like the birth of a grandchild, marriage of a child, a wedding anniversary, or a visit from a person important to them.

There seems to be a quality about some people, a personal characteristic that allows them some internal control over letting go of life or holding on to it a bit longer. That ability is not likely to be useful in prolonging life beyond the allotted life span, but it may be useful in allowing individuals to die a peaceful death. That internal control may be conditioned by society and culture. The meaning of death in the culture may provide the individual the opportunity to accept or reject an active role in the death process.

SUMMARY

People die within society, not apart from it. Values and attitudes toward death are taught and conditioned by the society in which one lives. Social conditions like sanitation and nutrition predispose one to health or illness. Whether a group of people chooses to confront death or deny it is determined at least in part by the mores of the whole society. Language and other symbols, such as art, literature, and drama, condition people to think of death in certain ways.

Death rates have changed through the years. Although there seems to be a finite number of years of life, the greatest number of deaths in any generation has risen from the time when most people who were born died in infancy, to a time when infection and plague decimated the population, to a time when most people have a reasonable expectation of dying in old age. For most of human history, it was reasonable to fight to achieve longer life because death was premature when compared to the standard of 85 years. Technologic death has been accepted because the technology used provided a reasonable hope of restoring the person to society. Now, however, prolongation of life as a societal goal is being reviewed, and the goal of a peaceful death reconsidered. This apparent conflict of goals has led to frequent, impassioned debate, a debate in which nurses should certainly take part.

REFERENCES

Callahan, D. (1993) Pursuing a peaceful death. In *The troubled dream of life: Living with mortality*. New York: Simon & Schuster.

Cassel, C. K., & Foley, K. M. (1998). *Principles for care of patients at end of life: An emerging concensus among the specialties of medicine* (p. 2). New York: The Milbank Memorial Fund.

Doyle, D., Hanks, G. W. C., & MacDonald, N. (Eds.). (1993). *Oxford textbook of palliative medicine*. Oxford: Oxford University Press.

Hamilton, D. (1991). Vital energy: The antebellum health movement. *Journal of Holistic Nursing, 9*(3), 10–19.

Kearl, M. C. (1989). *Endings: A sociology of death and dying*. New York: Oxford University Press.

Lancaster, H. O. (1990). *Expectations of life: A study in the demography, statistics, and history of world mortality*. New York: Springer-Verlag.

Riley, J. C. (1989). *Sickness, recovery and death: A history and forecast of ill health*. Iowa City, Iowa: University of Iowa Press.

U.S. Bureau of the Census. Statistical Abstracts of the U.S.: 1992 (Ed. 112, p. 76). Washington, DC.

Youngner, S. J. (1988). Who defines futility? *Journal of the American Medical Association, 260*, 2094–2095.

CHAPTER 3

Theories Related to Dying, Healing

THE USEFULNESS OF THEORY

Nursing practice is guided by theory. Relevant theory provides a framework that suggests to the practitioner what has happened, what to look for, how to measure an event, and what treatments or actions are most likely to yield some desirable outcome. Theories are not mutually exclusive. They may be used together if they use common terminology and concepts.

Theories are not always identified as theories. They are taught as a way of doing things, and they become patterns of behavior. An example is the nursing process. It is taught to almost all nursing students as a way of providing nursing care for all patients. Nurses learn to assess, plan, treat, and evaluate care. It becomes a standard, a pattern of behavior that nurses share in caring for patients.

Nursing theories are attempts by nurses to look at the theoretical foundations of the discipline of nursing. They may be based on an even larger theory, such as general systems theory from science or phenomenological theory from philosophy. Nursing theories are broad and can accommodate the addition of mid-range theories. Mid-range theories help focus on smaller areas of interest in the care of patients. They can be useful in further developing the way nurses address the care of grieving, dying patients and their families.

Different theorists have studied concepts and relationships of grief, families, culture, and self-transcendence. Grief theory aims to describe the grief process and to develop useful ways to help people resolve grief. It describes the significance of the resolution of grief in people's lives. Combining family theory and grief theory is useful in helping the family members to transcend grief in order to help the dying person while living their own lives. Self-transcendence as a theory focuses on an inner connectedness that helps move people toward peace and meaning in life.

GRIEF THEORY

Grief is a universal human experience. It is also intensely personal. Understanding what is universal and allowing the expression of what is personal help the nurse to plan sensitive, effective care for dying people and their families.

Definitions

Sometimes the term *grief* is used synonymously with loss, mourning, or bereavement. There are subtle differences (see Table 3-1). Grief is the internal sadness resulting from loss, and cannot be measured in time. Loss (of someone or something meaningful) precipitates the states of bereavement and mourning. Mourning is a connection with cultural rituals, acting out feelings of sadness. In some cultures, a young widow who

TABLE 3-1	Definitions of Terms Related to Grief
TERM	**DEFINITION**
Loss:	absence of someone or something meaningful.
Bereavement:	a response to the loss of something, or someone.
Mourning:	a feeling or expression of sorrow or sadness following loss.
Depression:	1) sadness gone awry. 2) A clinical diagnosis of an illness that sometimes follows significant loss. It can be treated successfully in most people. 3) A stage of grief in some theories that is normal if not prolonged.

is in mourning may wear black for a year following the death of her husband. The term *a period of mourning* may mean a variable period of time, perhaps a few months or a year, depending on the closeness of the bereaved to the one who died. Bereavement refers to a specific kind of loss, the death of a significant person in one's life.

Loss that results in grief may result from any life change. Losses occurring naturally in relation to life changes often include:

- divorce
- retirement
- moving
- unemployment
- amputation
- paralysis or other disability
- loss of sexual intimacy
- empty-nest syndrome
- aging

Losses that occur during a prolonged dying process include:

- loss of function
- loss of relationship
- loss of sexual intimacy
- loss of control

The grieving process that results from loss varies widely in intensity depending on the nature of what was lost, the unique reaction of the individual or group affected, past loss history, and the culture, subculture, and family system (Sunderland, 1993).

Grief, as a theory, links concepts into a whole fabric of ideas that help decide action. Grief theory has its origins in psychoanalytic theory (Freud, 1957); psychology (Caplan, 1974); pastoral care (Kushner, 1981); and medicine (Kübler-Ross, 1969; Lindemann, 1944). Grief studies by nurses became more common after the publication and popularization of the works of Kübler-Ross (who is not a nurse) on the stages of grief in the 1960s. Quint (1966) was one of the first nurses to study grief systematically. Both Quint and Kübler-Ross focused on grief associated with the loss of a loved one, not on grief related to the loss of goods, health, or other things.

There are a variety of theories that attempt to link concepts into a meaningful understanding of grief and to direct action. Some look at grief as reaction to loss; others as separation anxiety; still others as a function of attachment instincts (Sunderland, 1993, p. 27). Most nurses are familiar with developmental theory and find it to be a useful tool to understand grief and plan care. Some theorists discuss stage, some tasks, and some discuss phases.

Developmental Theory

Developmental theory classifies life into stages. Erickson's (1963) eight stages of life are well known for describing the tasks each individual should achieve before moving to the next stage, an ordered progression through life. Lindemann (1944) proposed the idea that grieving people enter a series of stages. Lindemann's stages represented five classes of symptoms that normal grieving people develop. Symptoms include somatic distress, preoccupation with the image of the deceased, guilt, hostility, and "loss of patterns of conduct" (a kind of restlessness and inability to concentrate). Lindemann's work is now considered a classic, though grief theory has developed in other directions.

The same idea of developmental stages was used by Kübler-Ross (1975) in her book *Death: The Final Stage of Growth*. Death is perceived as something to be achieved, another rung on a ladder. Such a theory allows one to contemplate a variety of philosophies relating to what happens after death. Kübler-Ross identified five stages that grieving people normally use to cope with their losses. Much earlier, Bowlby (1961) had noted four different stages of grieving. Their respective stages are compared in Table 3-2.

Developmental theorists point out that the stages they identify are not mutually exclusive. A grieving person may go back and forth between

TABLE 3-2	Comparison of Grief Stages			
STAGES 1		THROUGH		5
Kübler-Ross	Denial	Anger	Bargaining	Depression	Acceptance
Bowlby	Protest	Despair		Detachment	Resolution

them, often quite quickly. A grieving person may be denying the death of a loved one, but in only a few minutes become very angry about it. Or a person may begin to regain control, only to slip back into withdrawal on a subsequent day. Stages of grief are transient.

Characteristics of Grief

Cowles and Rodgers (1991) analyzed the nursing and medical literature to define grief. They defined grief as "a pervasive, highly individualized, dynamic process that often is discussed normatively within professional disciplines."

Grief is pervasive. It has the potential to affect every aspect of life. One can develop physical symptoms, such as inability to swallow, feeling of palpitations in the heart, hyperventilation, and others, as a response to grief. It can be hard to make decisions or to do the things one usually does. Thoughts, behaviors, and feelings are all affected. One tends to be preoccupied with the one who died (or is dying), cannot concentrate on what others may be saying, does not want to make choices, or makes choices without much thought. This intense kind of grief is termed *acute,* though it can recur long after the death.

Grief is also individualized. How people grieve depends on:

- the nature of their relationship with the one lost
- the presence of a support system
- previous losses in their lives
- religious and spiritual background
- cultural beliefs about how to grieve

No one grieves quite like anyone else and no one resolves grief like anyone else. The ability to use grief to reach a new level of experience is also variable.

Grief is dynamic. Cowles and Rodgers (1991) used the word *dynamic* to indicate the changing, moving nature of grief. They found little evidence of phases, but of feelings, thoughts, and sensations flowing back and forth. Grief seems to be viewed more as a process, as work to be done, as clusters of activity. Bowlby (1961) visualized a spiral figure that illustrated the progress of grief through life, in which each grief experience passed through the same behaviors and feelings as the previous grief experience. Although earlier theorists suggest a time period of six months to two years to move through the grief process, many now find that it may be limitless. Anniversaries of special times, including the loss itself, or special days like Memorial Day, may rekindle the emotions and revive grief (Hess, 1990).

Grief may be chronic. A young woman related the story of her father's chronic and terminal illness (Rosenberg, 1998), and described how chronic sorrow made its presence known in the life of the family. The father sobbed suddenly, for one of the few times in his life, in the presence of his children when he realized they may never see him again. He could not control his sudden outburst. Rosenberg similarly burst into tears several years later when she saw a favorite shirt of his in a garage sale. She pointed out that the family and her father also experienced moments of joy and laughter. Though one may be surprised by a sudden expression of grief a long time after the loss or bereavement, those moments are short and do not overshadow the moments of well-being. Those involved can "realize a transformation to a new level of health."

Grief is normative. That is, grief is defined by society and culture as normal, atypical, or pathological. The way a person responds to grief is given a value judgment by the group one lives with, according to the group's norms. This is particularly true in the professional disciplines. The hospital is a particular kind of environment. Immediately after the death of a loved one, family or friends are expected to make decisions about organ donation, or choice of funeral home, or whom to call first. If they cry, staff may be uncomfortable, but if they don't, they may risk being seen as cold or unfeeling.

Consequences of Grieving

People going through the dynamic process of grief in their own ways, but tied to their society by cultural mores, achieve two long-term consequences. They seem to develop a new reality and a new sense of self (identity). The new reality is that for the families there are new roles that do not include the deceased. There may also be new circumstances for the survivors, such as changed financial status or feeling less welcome at events for couples only. These new roles, which are forced on the survivors, cause survivors to think and act differently. In order to take on new roles, family members may need to learn to do new things, like managing finances. A new widow may learn to play bridge as a way to meet people. Inevitably, these changes force a change in how people think about themselves.

A bereaved person has choices. The new identity might include pride in accomplishing tasks or the refusal to consider a necessary change, which will lead to continued sadness and continued grieving. In American society, grieving too long is called *dysfunctional grieving*, thereby giving it the connotation of illness. The rationale for that is the inability to function appropriately in society. The consequences of grief for the dying person include the new reality and the new identity, but there is less time to achieve these things, and less energy. Hess (1990) described three clinical phases that occur between the time the dying person recognizes that death is imminent, and death itself. They are: (1) acute crisis; (2) chronic living–dying; and (3) terminal. These phases are pervasive, individual, and dynamic, as grief is for those who are not dying. They give some structure for caregivers to assist the dying individual with achievement of the tasks of dying.

In all phases, there should be a focus on creating an environment that accepts individual differences, supports the dying person in creating appropriate relationships with family and friends, and gives as much control over the living–dying process as the dying person is willing to take. The acute phase, in which the person and family and friends have learned of a fatal diagnosis, is an unstable period. Crisis intervention is commonly needed to help them refocus, deal with small losses as they occur, and support the cycle of denial and hope, which allows them to continue in a meaningful relationship for the time remaining.

Often, the chronic living–dying stage will continue for some time. The person who is dying must integrate care (e.g., chemotherapy, regular stress-tests, and so on) into an already full program of work, family, and social obligations. A priority must be placed on doing those things that are important to accomplish in the life span remaining, and to conserve energy and time. Decisions to take an active role in treatment, including the less traditional activities of massage, imagery, and meditation, should be advocated to the extent that they support hope and move a person toward hardiness. Continued evaluation and changes in the schedule of things to be done takes into account diminishing energy and ability. The same planning should be done to accomplish the resolution of psychological tasks and things the person wants to do before death. Family members often ask what they should do. It is important for them to understand that at times, the best thing to do is to *be*. Being requires the ability to sit quietly, perhaps hold hands or touch, and just share the same room. That may be what is needed at that moment. Relationships should be a priority. The ability to resolve an old argument with a parent, to leave a message for children, or to say good-bye in a meaningful way to a spouse allows the person to work toward a sense that life has had meaning.

The terminal phase may find the person drawing inward. Most tasks have been accomplished or abandoned. More physical support is required during this time, as well as time to be quiet. Friends and family may talk quietly, but not require much interaction with the dying one. Hope changes from a wish for remission or miracle cures to comfort with what is, an integration or acceptance of impending death.

FAMILY THEORY

Like grief theory, family theory provides guidance for nursing practice, in that everyone is a product of a family and an emotional system. Each individual is a part of a greater whole. Mr. Bower (Chapter 1) initially said he had no family. But he was a veteran and his compatriots were very much like his family. When any one of them died, all of them grieved.

The dying person grieves with family, and when death comes, the family left behind continues to grieve. The family often needs nursing support.

Additionally, family theory is important in the study of dying because families provide the support for a dying member. Families have the potential for helping the dying person, or making the dying more difficult. So, it is an important part of the nursing role to assess the potential for support by family, and the need they may have for intervention.

Types of Families

There are many types of families. Three family types have traditionally been identified. The family of origin is the one a person is born into (or enters into at a very early age), and includes mother, father, brothers, and sisters. This group is also the nuclear family for the parents. The nuclear family is the family of "marriage, parenthood, or procreation" (Friedman, 1986). It includes mother, father, and their children. The extended family includes those relationships by blood or marriage in the next level from the nuclear family. They are grandparents, aunts and uncles, and cousins.

There are many people who do not live in any of those types of families. Friedman (1986) defined family as "two or more people who are emotionally involved with each other and live in close geographical proximity." Using that definition, several other family types can be identified. Family forms include:

- single parent family
- kin network (living alone, near relatives)
- cohabitating couple
- commune
- homosexual union

The word *family*, when linked with other words, may give more definition to these structures. For example, the adoptive family may be a nuclear family, with one or more of the children having been adopted.

Family Theories

Like grief theory, family theory has its origins in psychoanalytic theory, psychology, sociology, and related disciplines. The Becvars (1988) began a history of family therapy in the 1930s and 1940s, citing such diverse contributors to the interdisciplinary approach as cybernetics and anthropology.

Family theory may be categorized as either a developmental theory or a systems theory, depending on the theorist. Interaction theory and structural/functional theory are also useful frameworks (see Table 3-3). The unit of analysis, or the focus of the theory, is the whole family. Individuals make up the family, and so are of interest in terms of how they relate within the family.

Developmental Family Theory

Developmental family theory views the family as having a life cycle. There are tasks the family does at different points in the cycle. Duvall (1977) formulated eight "core developmental tasks," which paralleled his family life cycle. The family begins with a marriage, expands through childbearing, preschool, school-age, teenagers, and launching. It then begins to contract through stages of middle-age and aging. The role of

TABLE 3-3	Approaches to Family Theory
APPROACH	FOCUS
Development	Family is a small group, progressing through identified stages over a life cycle.
Interactional	Family is a set of interacting personalities.
Structural/functional	Family is a social system that has characteristics of a small group and functions that serve both individual family members and society.
Systems	Family is an open social system that uses feedback for self-regulation, and individuals are subsystems that interact within the family and beyond the family.

each individual in the family is designed to achieve the tasks of the group. Family tasks include:

- provision of shelter and necessities, including health care
- allocation of resources
- determination of individual tasks (who does what)
- socialization
- establishment of ways of interacting
- child rearing
- community life
- developing family loyalties and values

The way in which family members react to grief is determined to a large extent by how each accomplishes the identified tasks. What they believe about health; how they socialize with each other, the extended family, and other people; and their values all give direction to their relationship with the person dying (or with themselves, if they are dying). Using a developmental framework in which to plan care for a grieving family, the nurse would assess which stage of development the family is in, knowing that grief is different at different stages in the family's life. A child's death would signal unfulfilled potential, unfinished tasks, while the death of the aged may be fulfillment of expectation. Affection may be available to some but not to other family members. Certain behaviors, like withdrawal, may be unacceptable in some, depending on their expected role. An eldest son may be expected to deliver the eulogy at his father's funeral, while his mother is free to cry.

When Duvall began his theory development, families were less complex, and generally thought of as nuclear families. Although Duvall's theory was a beginning, the changing nature of the American family meant that theorists began looking at families in different ways. Many tasks of families that Duvall identified continue to be relevant. For example, socialization, the provision of shelter, and the establishment of consistent values occur within the family structure, no matter what form a particular family may take. But child rearing for a childless couple or differentiation of tasks in a single adult home is only meaningful as it relates to the larger family, and family theories are moving away from developmental theories to other models. It is probably more efficient to view families in a different way than to try to trace the developmental stages for each of the forms of family that now exist.

Structural/Functional Family Theory

Friedman (1986) attempted to integrate family structure and function to create a useful model of family care. She identified four structural dimensions of family:

- role structure
- value systems
- communication processes
- power structure

Using the idea of outcomes of family structure as functions, she integrated five functions of families (affective function, or personality maintenance for individuals; socialization, primarily of the children; reproduction; economic function; and health care function). Each member of the family has a defined role and position. The role may be functional, such as the person who kisses the hurt and makes it well, or it may be based on position, for example, parent.

One way families relate is through family routines. Denham (1995) showed how family routines, defined as "day-to-day repetitive activities which occur within the family unit in a predictable manner," contribute to symbolic family representation, leading to family identity, individual identity, and social identity. Interruptions in family routines through loss and grief fundamentally disturbs the family identity and structure, and through that, all of society in some way.

When the loss of a family member is anticipated, the role of the dying person must be reassigned, and tasks redistributed. If this is done before the death occurs, the person dying may feel left out, devalued. Or the dying one may share in decisions and develop a feeling of continuity with the family even if absent. If the role is left unfilled, the family may suffer. Working out the new ways each family member must relate to other family members with sensitivity and compassion is a task of the family. They may require help in knowing when the dying family member is ready to give up the role or to accept help with it.

Family Systems Theory

Systems theory views families as social systems that are self-regulating. They identify their own boundaries by identifying those who are included in the family or with whom the family chooses to interact. Individuals are components of the system. Specific pathways of communication are required to maintain family health. Disruption such as a loss requires new channels of communication and affords the opportunity to create new ways of relating.

Two major concepts of family systems theory are feedback (communication) and adaptation. An open family (one that welcomes new ideas, actively problem solves, and interacts with the larger community) generally has established communication systems within the family and with the community. This gives access to support systems, means of expressing feelings, and outlets for emotions that are acceptable to the family. By contrast, a closed family is distrustful, controlling its members by force, and focused on predictability in relationships. Communication is by standard, proscribed means. A family that is too open does not filter or evaluate the information it receives and can become disorganized and chaotic. A family that is too closed does not receive enough information and cannot change.

Adaptation is seen as cyclical. The family strives for stability, for maintaining preferred patterns of behavior as long as possible because it helps to develop a feeling of security. But demands of the community and home environment occur, requiring change. For example, an adolescent begins to date. Perhaps the zoning laws change and the neighbors start to raise chickens. Or a loved one is diagnosed with an incurable disease. How the family responds to each of these events, how it adapts, depends on how it evaluates the information in terms of family values and goals, and patterns of communication and behavior it has developed over time.

Family systems theory has been developed into several specific forms of family therapy, all building upon the principles of systems. Three of the more useful theorists for nursing care are Virginia Satir, Salvador Minuchin, and Murray Bowen.

Grief and Family

Using the systems perspective, Walsh and McGoldrick (1991) identified two major tasks of people who are grieving. The first is "shared acknowledgment of the reality of death and shared experience of loss." The acknowledgment of death in a death-denying culture can pose real problems. If clear communication patterns have not been established within the family, and especially with the one who is dying, it may be difficult for the dying person to talk about death, to use the knowledge to finish his business and work toward a peaceful death. The family, too, may fail to use the time before the death occurs to prepare for the impending changes or say appropriate good-byes. Worse, according to Bowen (1976), they may become "stuck" in a pattern, unable to grow into new relationships after the death, reliving the death unknowingly at inappropriate times. For example, a parent who lost her mother at the age of 16, two years after she started dating, may treat her own daughter of 16 years as a 16 year old for several years in spite of the fact that her child is getting older and society expects change.

Family communication patterns may be functional or dysfunctional, and a careful assessment by the nurse to learn how information is shared in the family will help determine the need for nursing support. Bowen (1976) said that patterns in families persist for three to five generations. If some family members dominate communication patterns over two or three generations, establishing or changing patterns of communication after those persons die may require therapy for those who are left. Professionals in advanced practice nursing who specialize in communication patterns, grief work, or psychiatric nursing can help family members learn new ways to relate.

An interesting way of assessing patterns across generations is the use of genograms (see Figure 3-1). Genograms are pictorial representations of family relationships, and three to five generations can be included on

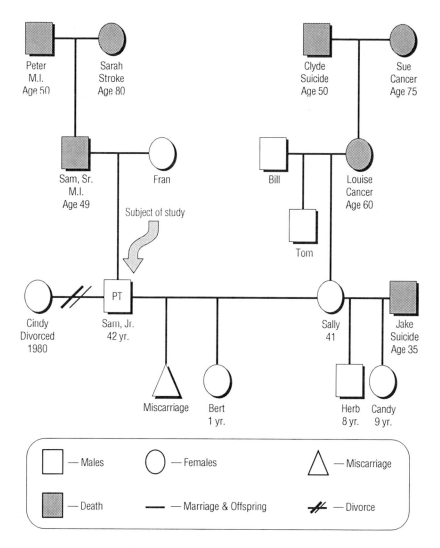

Figure 3-1 Three Generational Genogram

one form. Patterns of relationships, including how people died and at what age, major diseases, marital status of family members, including divorce, separation, singleness, and long-term marriage, are seen at a glance (McGoldrick & Gerson, 1985). Creating the genogram can be done with the dying person, with the family, or with both, and can help to begin a discussion about death and what it means to the family.

Figure 3-1 shows Sam, Jr. as the central person of interest. His father is dead, mother living. He is divorced from his first wife. His present wife had a previous marriage and was widowed. She had two children from that marriage who are now eight and nine years old. She and Sam, Jr. married and had a child. One other pregnancy ended in miscarriage. From the genogram, it is possible to detect other family information, like whether Sally's parents are alive, and the sex of Sam's children. Genograms are efficient ways of communicating a large amount of family information.

The second major task of grieving is "reorganization of the family system and reinvestment in other relationships and life pursuits" (Walsh and McGoldrick, 1991). Sometimes women who say they want to carry on the way their deceased spouse would want are not reorganizing or investing in new relationships. On the other hand, there is Mrs. J.

Mrs. J.

Mr. J. died in July. Mrs. J's mother died in August. Both of them had experienced long illnesses, during which Mrs. J. cared for them. She had grieved a lot. In September, Mrs. J. entered the hospital for an elective coronary artery bypass operation. The nurse knew that after the death of a spouse, some surviving spouses become depressed and even die. She asked Mrs. J. why she had made the decision to have the operation at this time. Mrs. J. replied that she had loved her husband very much. During the year she had cared for both him and her mother, she had developed cardiac symptoms, including angina pectoris. She, too, knew that it looked as if she might have a death wish following the deaths of her loved ones. After discussing it with her daughter, she had decided that her appropriate course of action was to get herself in the best possible physical condition so that she could get on with her life. This meant having surgery. She planned to learn to play bridge so that she could join a bridge club and meet people. And she wanted to enjoy her grandchildren. She was reinvesting in relationships, reorganizing her life. It was interesting to note that Mrs. J.'s mother had lost her husband at about the same age. She had joined the senior citizens' organization, gone on regular outings with others in the church group, and had become quite active in a social way for the rest of her life. Twelve years after the surgery, Mrs. J. is 82 years old and has a steady male friend with whom she enjoys travel, concerts, and parties.

Mrs. J. is an example of successful resolution of grief. She remembers her spouse on anniversaries, but has new relationships and new patterns of living. Her life has meaning to her. She is at peace. She believes that when it is her time to die, her life will have mattered.

CULTURE

Families are a part of culture (see Figure 3-2). Contemporary definitions of culture move beyond the traditional emphasis on race and ethnicity to include such variables as age (the culture of youth), economic status (the culture of poverty), and sexual orientation (gay culture). It is not uncommon to hear of a culture of homelessness, country club culture, and even women's culture. Rather than use the term culture as a modifier to define a group, more and more people are defining culture as a process (Barnes, Craig, & Chambers, 2000). Race and ethnicity contribute to cultural diversity and to values that determine, in part, one's goals and beliefs about health care and "a good death." But there are many other forms of culture that influence a patient's view of health and illness that must be considered by caregivers.

Currently, the U.S. population consists of 28.1% ethnic minorities and 7.9% whites or Anglo-Americans (U.S. Census Bureau, 1999). By the year 2050, minority groups (Asians, African Americans, and Hispanics) may nearly equal the current majority, at 48% (Norbeck, 1995). For people planning public policy and care for populations within the United States and around the world, understanding cultural diversity and caring for people in a culturally competent way is an imperative,

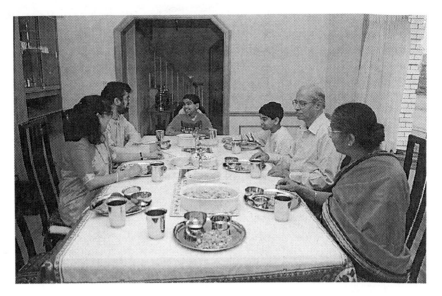

Figure 3-2 The family is often a vehicle by which cultural heritage is passed down to future generations.

a part of the care of the whole person. Meleis (1996) believed there is an urgency to develop scholarship and policies that will provide a foundation for the provision of culturally competent care. Many things drive this urgency. The changing of borders and countries' geography in all parts of the world contributes to the need for an understanding of values, beliefs, and goals across borders.

There is increasing diversity in relationships and lifestyles, such as marriages between traditional ethnic enemies, or gay couples. There are increasing population shifts due to immigration or war. And there is a backlash by people struggling to establish or maintain traditional identities and still have access to health care services and other social services. An example is the demonstration of "gay pride" in New York and San Francisco in the United States and Sydney, Australia.

Traditionally, nurses and other health care providers have written about being culturally sensitive, and taking into account a person's culture when giving care. But little action was devoted to learning or teaching what those cultures required in terms of end-of-life decisions beyond care of the body, dietary restrictions, and certain rites, such as anointing and burial customs. Goals for a good death were thought to be universal, or at least treated that way, if they were thought about. In Papua New Guinea, a man brought his wife into the hospital for treatment of a severe abdominal infection. When she began to have a strong odor because of the infection, the man prepared to take her home. When the nurse asked why he wanted to take her home before she was cured, he replied in his own language that she had begun to smell, so she must be dead. He was going to bury her even though she was still talking. In many other countries, this would be a criminal act. The strong odor had a different meaning for this man and his culture, and knowledge of that meaning would have helped the nurse plan care differently. Care could have included measures to limit the odor, or an explanation to the husband of the meaning of the odor during the care process so he would have a new context for the information. Instead, her first thought was to protect the woman from being buried alive.

There has been a shift in the thinking of nurses regarding culture. Leininger (1978, 1991, 1998) first introduced the idea that nursing care necessarily must be delivered with a cultural awareness, and developed a theory of transcultural nursing. Nursing as a profession respects differences between people and attempts to incorporate different values into care giving. This evolved into a variety of definitions related to culture and care giving.

- cultural awareness: recognizing differences in values, beliefs, and behaviors
- cultural diversity: differences in values, behaviors, and attitudes based on group membership and usually related to race or ethnicity
- cultural sensitivity: an awareness that the patient may have values, behaviors, and attitudes different from the nurse, and a willingness to explore these differences
- cultural competence: the ability to work effectively within a culture; a process

The National Academy of Nursing expert panel on culturally competent care has developed a more formal definition: "care that takes into account issues related to diversity, marginalization, and vulnerability due to culture, race, gender and sexual orientation. This care is guided by nursing theories, models, and/or research principles. . . . It is also care that is provided within the historical and 'dailiness' context of clients" (Meleis, Isenberg, Koerner, Lacey, & Stern, 1995, p. 4). Barnes, et. al. (2000), also believed that "knowledge is not enough, but that cultural experience and an ability to incorporate cultural knowledge into relevant client care are needed."

For many people of color, only care delivered by someone raised in the culture, or working with someone in the culture, is appropriate. But studies illustrate some universalities of culture in regard to health care. For example, Pollack (1999), reviewed studies done in the United States using the Health Related Hardiness Scale. She found that there was "empirical support that the presence of the health-related hardiness characteristic facilitates health promotion as well as promotes adaptation to health problems and other stressors in adults from different ethnic populations." Validation of hardiness as a universal health-related factor in other countries and languages is currently being done. How hardiness manifests itself in the different ethnic groups, and presumably different cultures as a whole, is likely to be different. Fear of death or of the process of death seems to be a universal factor in all cultures, though managed in different ways. The call for scholarship to define care needs at the end of life is a call to determine the universalities and the specifics that make care consistent with the patients' values and goals.

Cultural competence, as a process, requires a lifelong commitment to increasing cultural competence (Wenger, 1999). For some, this means one must actively search for cultural experiences that expand one's world view (Meleis, 1999). For others, the practical outcome of working effectively within a culture is proof of the cultural competence of a health care provider (Campinha-Bacote, 1999). Rabbia, a dying person (de Mange, 1998), illustrates this beautifully. She was an African American Muslim woman. The care the professional nurse gave reflected high standards, meeting physical needs, offering professional touch, allowing the family to stay and help. But she also pulled the sheets down over the woman's body to inspect her body, was somewhat rough (according to Rabbia), and had to be reminded to put a scarf over Rabbia's head after death, as the family was returning to the room to spend time with her. The Muslim women who also cared for her were different. They protected Rabbia's modesty at all times, and kept her scarf on her head as is customary, even after death. They recited the prayers with which she was comfortable, while she was dying and after death until she was buried. Preparation of her body was not just washing, but a perfuming and anointing-type of ceremony. They talked to her until she was buried, describing each procedure to the now dead woman.

Purnell and Paulanka (1998) developed a theory of cultural competence illustrated by a continuum, showing how a person progresses in a nonlinear fashion from incompetence to competence. One moves through the following stages:

- no awareness of one's lack of knowledge of cultural issues (unconscious incompetence)

- becoming aware of one's lack of knowledge of cultural issues (conscious incompetence)

- learning about the relevant cultural issues in a person's care (conscious competence)

- automatically giving culturally congruent care to persons of diverse cultures (unconscious competence)

The active journey to achieve cultural competence is aided by both individual change and environmental, or organizational change. Using the continuum, it is easy to see that the first step is consciousness raising, or becoming aware of the need to understand another's culture. Some counsel that this is best done by having an experience in another country or culture different from your own. That may be part of the reason for the increasing numbers of courses in transcultural nursing that include such an experience. But there are other means to accomplish an increasing awareness of cultural issues. Working consistently with diverse populations is one. Deliberately seeking out opportunities to meet with people from other cultures instead of avoiding them indicates one has moved a step closer to cultural competence. Talking about cultural issues that are at odds with your own and identifying people with whom you can share feelings about those differences can help. Reevaluating your care in the light of what you have learned provides the basis on which you can improve your care.

Organizations and institutions are responsible for providing an environment that supports culturally competent care. De Mange (1998) the author of Rabbia's story gave some suggestions:

- incorporate patients' cultural values and beliefs about death into patient care standards
- encourage discussion and educational opportunities for nurses and other health care providers about beliefs and conflicts in caring for the dying
- hold open discussions with appropriate professionals about ethical and legal issues
- include reference materials on cultural perspectives on death in the institutions' libraries
- hold open forums with representatives of various religious and cultural organizations
- allow adequate time for giving care in a culturally competent manner
- develop mentorships for inexperienced nurses caring for dying people

Culturally competent care does not just happen. Even within one's own culture, there is a variety of beliefs about death held by family and society. Becoming culturally competent is a requirement of holistic care.

SELF-TRANSCENDENCE

Theories of self-transcendence are based on the assumption that a sense of connectedness between the innermost sense of self and the environment is a universal human characteristic. Self-transcendence is an expansion of one's conceptual boundaries inwardly through introspective activities, outwardly through concerns about others' welfare, and temporally by integrating perceptions of one's past and future to enhance the present (Reed, 1991a).

This expansion of self-boundaries orients one to a broadened sense of purpose in life. It defines meaning in life.

Self-transcendence has been studied largely in association with end-of-life issues. At the end of life, concern about meaning is a recurrent theme, and many people confronting death ask questions starting with *why* for this reason. Frankl (1963), himself a camp survivor, studied other concentration camp survivors to discover why some people who seemed weak survived when others, who seemed much stronger, did not. He found that those who survived found purpose and meaning even in the camp situation. For Frankl, one transcends either toward other people or toward meaning. One does so in one of three ways. It may be by creativity (either in family or in creative works). It may be by receptivity to others and the environment. Or it may be by developing an attitude of acceptance when a situation cannot be changed (Coward, 1991). Vaughn (1985) presented the following words to describe the self-transcendent person: compassionate, wise, receptive, creative, open, connected, intuitive, and spiritual. The person has moved beyond self-concern without devaluing self. Reaching out to others, the self-transcendent person develops a greater sense of meaning and purpose by helping others. Many peer support groups are led by people who find meaning in helping others cope with the same diagnoses and treatments they have had.

Self-transcendence has been linked with less depression, self-neglect, and feelings of hopelessness (Reed, 1991b). Self-transcendent people have a greater sense of well-being and the ability to cope with grief (Coward, 1991). Part of the coping ability is related to the willingness of self-transcendent people to accept and to give support. Part of it also has to do with the ability of the self-transcendent person to live in the present rather than in the past. A self-transcendent person may see death as a natural part of life.

It is unrealistic to expect all dying patients to achieve self-transcendence.

Yet, all people approaching the end of life should be supported in searching for meaning or connectedness. Finding meaning and connecting with others makes grieving less difficult. One learns to turn an experience that is potentially devastating into a reason for hope. Sometimes transcendence occurs in a particularly short period (the *transcendent moment*), and great and lasting joy may be a component of the experience. This is often true of the person who achieves transcendence as a spiritual experience. Certainly the self-transcendent person achieves peace.

Caregiving is a difficult experience, especially if it is prolonged. Many theorists have suggested that people have the ability to make meaning of difficult life experience, to reach beyond self. The popular admonition, "if life gives you lemons, make lemonade," reflects this

Mr. Bower, Luke, and the Nurse

Mr. Bower, a patient known for his rather stern manner, occupied a room across the hall from another patient, Luke. Luke was dying. He needed oxygen to breathe more easily, but oxygen was available in the rooms on the other side of the hallway, not in his room. Getting tanks of oxygen took time. Although it was 3 A.M., Mr. Bower saw the activity and preparations and asked what was happening. He offered to change rooms so that Luke could have the oxygen immediately. The change was made. After all the interventions that could be given had been given, Luke died at 7 A.M. Through all the frantic activity, Mr. Bower sat quietly by Luke's side. The nurse had to do the many tasks of caring for the dead that hospitals prescribe, so she was very late getting off duty. Mr. Bower walked the nurse to the elevator although he was in some pain. As she thanked him for his willingness to give up his room for the comfort of another, he said, "I sure hope you are there when it is my turn to go. You give a guy a fighting chance!" This gruff man had recognized the nurse's need for support and connected with her by acknowledging her competence and willingness to help.

notion. However, using this kind of statement with one who is deeply distressed denies the person's feelings. The use of such platitudes is not helpful. Acton and Wright (2000) believed that caregivers who move toward transcendence move away from isolation, loss, and hopelessness toward understanding, love, and healing.

Measures to help people achieve self-transcendence build on the need to look inward, the need to connect (with family as well as others), and the need for a sense of timelessness. Life review, for example, helps a person to look at life, see that it was unique and meaningful, remember those who are loved, and realize that a place in history is reserved. Nursing measures to promote self-transcendence are included in Chapter 7.

SUMMARY

Theories of grief, families, and transcendence provide direction for nursing care of the dying and their families. Knowing what patterns of behavior to expect from the dying patient and family members, and the patterns the family uses for coping and relating to each other help the nurse assess needs and determine strategies to meet those needs.

Self-transcendence is a sense of connecting inwardly to the deepest sense of self and outwardly in the form of relationships with others. Achieving self-transcendence toward the end of life helps a person see that life has meaning. The realization of meaning in life helps one to live each moment fully, capable of joy and peace in spite of impending death.

REFERENCES

Acton, G. J., & Wright, K. B. (2000). Self-transcendence and family caregivers of adults with dementia. *Journal of Holistic Nursing, 18*(2), 143–158.

Barnes, D. M., Craig, K. K., & Chambers, K. B. (2000). A review of the concept of culture in holistic nursing literature. *Journal of Holistic Nursing, 18*(3), 207–221.

Becvar, D. S., & Becvar, R. J. (1988). *Family therapy: A systemic integration.* Boston: Allyn and Bacon.

Bowen, M. (1976). Family reaction to death. In P. Guerin (Ed.), *Family therapy.* New York: Gardner.

Bowlby, J. (1961). Process of mourning. *International Journal of Psychoanalysis, 42,* 317.

Campinha-Bacote, J. (1999). A model and instrument for addressing cultural competence in health care. *Journal of Nursing Education, 38*(5), 203–207.

Caplan, G. (1974). Foreward. In I. Glick, R. Weiss, & C. Parkes (Eds.), *The first year of bereavement* (pp. vi–xi). New York: Wiley.

Coward, D. (1991). Self-transcendence and emotional well-being in women with advanced breast cancer. *Oncology Nursing Forum, 18*(5), 857–863.

Cowles, K. V., & Rodgers, B. L. (1991). The concept of grief: A foundation for nursing research and practice. *Research in Nursing and Health, 14,* 119–127.

de Mange, E. P. (1998). The story of Rabbia, a dying person. *Holistic Nursing Practice, 13*(1), 76–81.

Denham, S. A. (1995). Family routines: A construct for considering family health. *Holistic Nursing Practice, 9*(4), 11–23.

Duvall, E. M. (1977). *Marriage and family development.* Philadelphia: Lippincott.

Erickson, E. (1963). *Childhood and society.* New York: W.W. Norton & Co., Inc.

Frankl, V. (1963, ©1959). *Man's search for meaning* (3rd ed.). New York: Simon & Schuster.

Freud, S. (1957). Mourning and melancholia. In J. Strachey (Ed. and Trans.), *The standard edition of the complete psychological works of Sigmund Freud* (vol. 14, pp. 243–258). London: Hogarth Press.

Friedman, M. M. (1986). *Family nursing: Theory and assessment* (2nd ed.). Norwalk, CT: Appleton-Century-Crofts.

Hess, P. (1990). Loss, grief and dying. In P. Beare & J. L. Myers (Eds.), *Principles and practice of adult health nursing.* St. Louis, MO: C.V. Mosby, Co.

Kübler-Ross, E. (1969). *On death and dying.* New York: Macmillan.

Kübler-Ross, E. (1975). *Death: The final stage of growth.* Englewood Cliffs, NJ: Prentice Hall.

Kushner, H. S. (1981). *When bad things happen to good people.* New York: Schocken Books.

Leininger, M. (1978). Transcultural nursing theories and research approaches. In M. Leininger (Ed.), *Transcultural nursing: Concepts, theories, and practices.* New York: Wiley.

Leininger, M. (1991). *Culture care diversity and universality: A theory of nursing.* New York: National League for Nursing.

Leininger, M. (1998). Special research report: Dominant culture care meanings and practice findings from Leininger's theory. *Journal of Transcultural Nursing, 9*(2), 45–48.

Lindemann, E. (1944). Symptomatology and management of acute grief. *American Journal of Psychiatry, 101,* 141–148.

Meleis, A. I. (1996). Culturally competent scholarship: Substance and rigor. *Advances in Nursing Science, 19*(2), 11–16.

Meleis, A. I. (1999). Culturally competent care. *Journal of Transcultural Nursing, 10*(1), 12.

Meleis, A. I., Isenberg, M., Koerner, J. E., Lacey, B., & Stern, P. (1995). *Marginalization and culturally competent health care: Issues in knowledge development* (Monograph). New York. American Academy of Nursing Press.

McGoldrick, M., & Gerson, R. (1985). *Genograms in family assessment.* New York: W.W. Norton & Co.

Norbeck, J. (1995). Who is the consumer? Shaping nursing programs to meet emerging needs. *Journal of Professional Nursing, 11*(6), 325–331.

Pollack, S. E. (1999). Health-related hardiness with different ethnic populations. *Holistic Nursing Practice, 13*(3), 1–10.

Purnell, L. D., & Paulanka, B. J. (1998). *Transcultural health care: A culturally competent approach.* Philadelphia: F.A. Davis.

Quint, J. (1966). Awareness of death and the nurse's composure. *Nursing Research, 15,* 49–55.

Reed, P. (1991a). Self-transcendence and mental health in oldest-old adults. *Nursing Research, 40*(1), 5–11.

Reed, P. (1991b). Toward a nursing theory of self-transcendence: Deductive reformulation using developmental theories. *Advances in Nursing Science, 33*(4), 64–77.

Rosenberg, C. (1998). A father's chronic sorrow: A daughter's perspective. *Journal of Holistic Nursing, 16*(3), 399–404.

Sunderland, R. (1993). *Getting through grief: Caregiving by congregations.* Nashville, TN: Abingdon Press.

U.S. Census Bureau (1999). Population Estimates. Washington, DC: Author www.census.gov/population/estimates/nation/intfile3-1.txt.

Vaughn, F. (1985). Discovering transpersonal identity. *Journal of Humanistic Psychology, 25*(3), 13–38.

Walsh, F., & McGoldrick, M. (1991). *Living beyond loss: Death in the family.* New York: W.W. Norton & Co.

Wenger, A. F. Z. (1999). Cultural openness: Intrinsic to human care. *Journal of Transcultural Nursing, 10*(1), 10.

PART
II

Comfort of the Dying Individual

CHAPTER 4

Goals for Comfort in Dying

COMFORT DEFINED

Palliative care requires that caregivers strive to help the dying person be comfortable, even in the dying process. To strive for comfort is more than to strive to relieve pain. The goal of providing comfort and reducing discomfort for the dying person is to enable that person to live fully and satisfyingly until death occurs.

Discomfort comes from many sources. The inability to sleep, difficulty in movement, shattered dreams, and changing family roles and relationships are among the many sources of discomfort. Each of these discomforts affects the quality of a person's life.

Comfort is a multidimensional concept, meaning different things to different people. Comfort is positive and is experienced right now. It is a whole person attribute, meaning that the absence of comfort in one part of a person's existence causes the whole individual to be uncomfortable. It is not just a portion of the body, the emotions, or the spirit that suffers.

Kolcaba (1991, 1992) based her definition of comfort on patient needs. The intensity of comfort needs can be thought of as a continuum, ranging from relief on one end, through ease, and to transcendence on the other end. When a need is met, the person experiences relief. Ease occurs if the need is met and the person feels a sense of calm or serenity as a result. Transcendence occurs when the person is able to rise above negative circumstances like pain and achieve a sense of quality in life or meaning in being alive, in spite of problems. This idea of the transcendence, like the definition in Chapter 3, requires the individual to reach inside himself and see the connection of self to something beyond self. Kolcaba defines comfort as "the immediate experience of having met basic human needs for relief, ease, and transcendence."

There are four kinds of internal or external comfort needs. They are

1. physical needs, or bodily sensations
2. psychospiritual, a dimension that includes awareness of self and a sense of meaning in life
3. environment, the context in which a person lives, including light, noise, odor, temperature
4. social, referring to relationships (Kolcaba, 1992)

Meeting basic human needs for comfort in the dying patient may include care within any of these four areas or any combination of them. Eliminating a noxious odor or providing a blanket changes the environment, and may provide relief or move a person into a state of ease, a higher level of comfort.

The provision of comfort has been a nursing tradition and value since Nightingale. Obviously, comfort is more than an absence of pain or absence of discomfort. Relief, as defined earlier, is closely related to the absence of pain or discomfort, but achievement of a feeling of ease and transcendence requires that the nurse's role include those measures that improve the patient's sense of well-being and quality of life. When setting goals for patient care, it is useful to consider both comfort and quality of life as indicators of the effectiveness of care.

QUALITY OF LIFE

Quality of life has been defined as psychological, physical, social/interpersonal, and financial/material well-being (Padilla, Grant, & Ferrell, 1992). Table 4-1 illustrates how closely Kolcaba's degrees of comfort needs and Padilla's components of quality of life agree. Quality of life is clearly affected by a person's level of comfort.

TABLE 4-1	Comfort and Quality of Life	
COMFORT*	**QUALITY OF LIFE****	
Physical	Physical	
Psychospiritual	Psychological	
Environment	Financial/material	
Social	Social/interpersonal	
*Kolcaba		
**Padilla et al.		

Although these theorists described areas of life that must be considered when assisting patients to achieve a sense of well-being, others have suggested that it is more complicated to decide what quality of life means. One view is that there is a gap between patient expectations of life and the reality of the situation. For example, the athlete with multiple sclerosis may expect to compete again, but the physical situation prohibits the same kind of competition as before. Quality of life in this scenario may depend on the size of the gap between the patient's expectation and the reality (Calman, 1984). The smaller the gap between expectation and reality, the greater the quality of life.

Building on that idea, a second view considers the possibility of reorganizing the strengths of an individual to achieve a new balance of mind and body, allowing a person to function at a new level. The individual achieves a different but acceptable way of living. Thus, she learns to cope with the loss of vital capacity of the lungs by walking more slowly or going out less frequently. Quality of life depends upon a person's ability to reorganize goals and abilities so that they balance.

Another view is based on the idea of a trade-off: probable length of life versus personal loss of some specific function. In one study, firefighters were more likely to choose to undergo a laryngectomy, which they were told would mean longer life, but without a voice, than businesspeople. The businesspeople felt the quality of life without a voice was unacceptable (McNeil, Weichselbaum, & Pauker, 1981). This illustrates how individual the idea of quality of life is. Comfortable, satisfying living for anyone, including the dying patient, must be evaluated by that person.

One longtime AIDS survivor credits his survival to having the financial resources to manage his environment. In addition to working with his traditional health care team, with whom he has an excellent relationship, he is able to create a peaceful, beautiful space in his backyard, growing roses and other flowers for color and enjoyment. He discusses alternative medical treatment with a variety of people he trusts, including his nurses. He chooses to stay out of crowds, limiting his risk of contracting contagious diseases. He regularly plans and gets comfort treatments, which he identifies as massage, Therapeutic Touch, and herbal treatments. His physician is fully aware of his self-medication with herbs and other over-the-counter medications, and supports his choices. He has many friends. It has been more than eight years since his first fevers were diagnosed as AIDS. His T-lymphocyte levels and other measures of potential decline have not changed, though he has had bouts of recurrent fevers and splenomegaly, requiring a splenectomy. He focuses on living a life in which he can be comfortable in each area of his life. It is his full-time job. His retirement income makes much of that possible.

This survivor is an example of a person using resources to live well. Although not all patients have such resources, most have some choices to make about their environment. Assessment of the patient's ability to identify and create an appropriate environment in which living well is possible is a part of the nursing assessment.

ASSESSMENT

Assessment helps to identify problems and makes it possible to plan to address them. Spending time doing an assessment has the added benefit of establishing trust between the health care provider and the patient. Areas of quality of life that are important to assess in people who are ill include physical, emotional, spiritual and social function; and symptoms of disease or side effects of treatment (Doyle, Hanks, & MacDonald, 1993) (see Table 4-2). It is important to get a list of all the doctors

TABLE 4-2	Assessment Components

A complete history of the illness
       Chronological history of illness development
       History of treatments accepted
       Present symptoms
       Methods the patient uses to control them
Physical examination
Social history
       Occupation
       Family history
       Conditions at home
       Caregivers
       Social groups
       Participation in religious organizations
Functional assessment

involved in care and to know who is coordinating care. It is also important to find out what others are involved in the multidisciplinary care team, such as social workers, clergy, and therapists. There are specific forms to be used to assess individual problems, such as pain or mobility, which are discussed later.

Functional assessment helps identify how well a person is coping with and living in a personal environment. Discomfort of any kind limits a person's abilities to control a setting, to achieve a set of aims, or to enjoy life. The individual making treatment decisions will make those decisions based on expected ability to function, ability to rebalance her strengths, satisfaction with the course of action, and available resources.

The Dartmouth COOP Functional Assessment tool (1994; Nelson, Wasson, Johnson, & Hays, 1996) is a short tool that can be used by clinicians each time the patient comes to the office. Its purpose is to determine if a change in functional status, like movement, has occurred. For patients who see the primary care professional regularly, but only for a short visit, it can be very useful in planning care. It takes only a minute or two to be completed, is valid for literate or illiterate clients, and can give direction for care because it documents improvement or decline. A statement is read to the client, like "During the past 2 weeks what was the hardest physical activity you could do for at least 2 minutes?" (Dartmouth COOP Project, 1994). The client then points to one of several stick figures engaged in activity from running to standing still. Nine scales are included in the format.

Other scales for functional or performance status include Karnofsky's Performance Status Scale, the New York Heart Association Functional Classification, and Reisberg's Functional Assessment strategy. These assessment forms are available in *Hospice Care* (1998). They are recommended by hospice organizations to determine prognosis and suitability for hospice care.

One of the earliest and still most comprehensive guides available for functional assessment was developed for the assessment of the elderly. The OARS Multidimensional Functional Assessment Questionnaire, developed at Duke University, is divided into two sections, the first related to individual functioning, and the second identifying the utilization of services. Each section takes about 35 minutes to complete.

Table 4-3 lists the topics covered in the OARS guide. This kind of form is useful because it is comprehensive, has been widely published (so is available), and gives enough information about what a person needs to be helpful in planning care. Based on the information, a nurse can determine which areas require further assessment. For example, a patient with a history of frequent falls may need to have his home assessed for hazards such as loose rugs, lack of support rails or bars in the bathroom, or dark areas of the house. These things become a problem for the patient at home who has medications that cause changes in sensorium and balance, or who has mobility problems and needs to hold on to handrails. Families may think of these things as elders become more frail, but they may not think of them when younger family members are sick and become frail. A major reason for doing a complete functional assessment is to prevent problems that interfere with maintaining the highest quality of life possible for as long as possible for the person who is dying.

Functional and hazards assessments are repeated as the patient's condition changes. Increasing frailty, dementia and confusion, and discom-

TABLE 4-3	Topics in OARS Functional Assessment

Personal:

Mental status	Living situation
Relationships	Economic resources
Physical health	Mobility
Sleep patterns	Activities of daily living

Services:

Transportation	Social/recreational services
Employment services	Educational services
Supervision	Placement services
Housekeeper services	Meal preparation
Legal, protective	Overall evaluation

Care required, by category:

Nursing
Pharmacy
Physical therapy
Psychiatric
Social work

Source: Duke University Center for the Study of Aging, 1975.

fort may require changes in care. For example, a patient who uses public transportation to visit the doctor's office may be required to step 18 inches up from the ground to the bus step. If that becomes impossible, other transportation arrangements may need to be made for doctor's visits. Changed plans might include being driven by family or friends, having home nursing services so that fewer visits are required to the doctor's office, or beginning to investigate hospice services or long-term care facilities for placement. Functional assessments that are used to plan ahead relieve the fear and the concern patient and family have when the situation requires change. Transition has been thought out, resources brought to the problem, and crisis avoided.

COMFORT FOR THE WHOLE PERSON

There are several ways of caring for individuals that help them deal with discomfort. They include the use of presence, surveillance and safety, providing choice, and care of the environment.

Presence

The concept of presence is a prerequisite to providing comfort that leads to the achievement of an improved quality of life. Hines (1987, p. 18) defined presence as "a mode of being available in a situation with the wholeness of one's unique individual being; a process resulting in an exchange of authentic meaningful awareness and essence linking and . . . ultimate realization of human potential." When two people are in a healing relationship, the aim is to produce a feeling of well-being, comfort, and growth. The nurse often shares this feeling with the patient. The patient usually is better able to cope as a result of the general feeling of comfort.

Characteristics of a relationship in which there is presence include: spending time together; a nonjudgmental, caring relationship; verbal and nonverbal communication; identification of the encounter as meaningful; connectedness—being open and honest in the relationship; and something Hines terms *sustaining memory*. Sustaining memory "involves presence in absence and the memorable impression and enduring impact made between individuals in the situation that affords comfort" (Hines, 1992; Pettigrew, 1988). For the dying person, this may be the recognition that "my life matters to this nurse." Mr. Bower's nurse has a sustaining memory of him, and he knew that he would be remembered after his death.

When two people connect in a healing relationship, the patient feels that she has been heard (see Figure 4-1). That is, the nurse or caregiver recognizes what the patient is saying, and trusts that the patient has knowledge of changes occurring in the body. The nurse does not tell the patient what to do, but fits care into the patient's context, or understanding. Patients who feel cared for feel more comfortable. They list several reasons for that feeling. Generally, feeling safe is a part of the comfort. The sense that someone understands their description of the problem

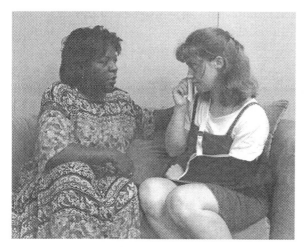

Figure 4-1
Nurse comforts patient
with presence.

and is monitoring it is a part of this feeling of safety. Providing information and demonstrating professional skills also help the patient feel safer.

Surveillance and Safety

A nurse who approaches the bedside of a sick person in an Intensive Care
Unit (ICU) and briefly chats with the patient before leaving may be perceived as monitoring the person if, while chatting, the nurse's eyes rest
briefly on each of the telemonitoring devices, each tube that drips, each
screen that gives information. The patient realizes that the eye movements of the nurse are a part of surveillance. Nurses who are experienced
and competent in their field are usually able to combine surveillance
with conversation. The conversation may be related to other assessment
parameters, such as symptoms experience or family changes, or the conversation may be unrelated to the patient's condition. A social experience
is also a patient need. Presence forms the matrix of the whole interaction,
and the feeling of safety and comfort is the outcome.

Choice

Another attribute of a relationship in which the patient can feel comfortable, cared for, and safe is the provision for autonomy. Recognizing the
individual experience of the patient, giving the patient choices regarding

care, and assistance with pain are all things patients have identified as essential to feeling cared for (Brown, 1986). If a relationship in which the dying patient feels cared for has been established, the patient is more willing to give control of care to others when strength and the will to make decisions diminishes. There is no need to expend energy consciously monitoring the care being given to him. The relationship is built on a trust that caregivers will respect his wishes and that the care given will be in harmony with his desires. The autonomy in this case is the ability to make a choice to continue to monitor care, or to spend energy on relationships, or to become introspective and self-focused. Trust that another person will carry out the patient's care in the preferred ways frees him to make real choices at the end of life.

Environment

Comfort for the whole person also includes care of the environment. Noxious odors, jarring noises, inappropriate lighting, crumbs in the bedclothes, absence of touch in one's life are all things that lead to discomfort. Therapeutic uses of aromas, music, touch, and other environmental components will be discussed separately.

The general principle guiding environmental care for the dying patient is to be sure that everything in the environment enhances the person's ability to use all senses. For example, lighting should be bright enough to see all hazards, such as things left on the floor or coffee tables in the path, and things that make life joyful, such as children or flowers, should be present. Music should not be so loud as to interfere with hearing other sounds, such as the doorbell or a conversation. Wrinkles in bedclothes can interfere with a person's sensations of developing skin breakdown because the wrinkles are annoying, and it is hard to differentiate them from a sore. It is important to have people in the environment. If a choice must be made between people in the environment and institutional policy or rules, the patient's goals and wishes are the guiding principles. For example, if a bone marrow transplant recipient is clearly dying, but the unit does not allow children to visit because of potential infection, the solution to the dilemma (to let the patient's children visit or not) should be made based on the patient's goals of how she wishes to die. Does she care about the potential for infection? Is she fighting for every moment of life that she can have? Or would the presence of her children be comforting, allowing her to let go of this world peacefully? Appropriate environmental control requires knowledge of the patient's goals for the end of life.

SPECIFIC AREAS OF COMFORT NEEDS

Sleep

A good night's sleep is a wonderful gift of nature. Although scientists continue to try to analyze the many specific results of adequate sleep, every person can understand sleep as a restorative process. There is a reciprocal relation between sleep and comfort. Lack of sleep leads to discomfort, and discomfort results in lack of sleep. Those treatments that lead to comfort are a prerequisite for helping the patient into restorative, restful sleep.

Fear of falling asleep is a real problem for some people. Shakespeare's "to sleep, perchance to dream; ay there's the rub" is only one of many literary references to the human condition of fear of falling asleep because of nightmares or dreams. Some people fear they may not waken. Dying people sometimes lay awake for hours, imagining all sorts of terrors that might accompany the end of their lives. Their anxiety is accompanied by perspiration, tense muscles, rapid respirations, and other physiologic symptoms of anxiety that reinforce their fears of a worsening condition. Such symptoms often exacerbate the symptoms of illness, such as pain. The next day finds them unrestored, with less energy to spend on living life.

A patient who is having difficulty sleeping may have one of a number of sleep disorders. However, if the sleep problems developed only after the life-threatening illness developed, it is likely that they are related to factors such as:

- symptoms, like pain or nausea
- intense emotion, like anger or fear

- social problems with family, job, or money
- unfamiliar environment, including a strange bed or lights
- medications or substances like alcohol or caffeine

Because dying people often experience more than one of these factors, sleep disruption is a common and very real problem for many dying patients. Avoiding as many of the factors that contribute to sleep deprivation as possible is an important part of care.

Insomnia is defined in general as a subjective complaint of poor sleep. It is subjective because no one can determine for another whether the amount or quality of the sleep cycle is adequate. Some people normally sleep only a few hours; others sleep eight, nine, or ten hours. Rhythms of sleep vary, with some people falling asleep after midnight and waking quite refreshed seven or eight hours later. Others cannot stay awake after 9:00 P.M. Changing these patterns to fit a hospital schedule can contribute to a feeling of daytime fatigue and broken sleep. Dying people often complain of poor sleep because they have been unable to maintain their natural patterns of sleep.

Poor sleep may be divided into two parts: the inability to fall asleep, and the inability to stay asleep. An unfamiliar bed or pain at bedtime is likely to make it difficult for the patient to go to sleep. But medications or drugs, including alcohol, are more likely to cause early awakenings. Avoiding alcohol after 6:00 P.M. or rescheduling medication may be all that is required.

Some sleeplessness is concurrent with a disease, but not a part of it. For example, a menopausal woman may suffer several awakenings at night related to hot flashes. If the treatment for her illness does not prohibit the use of hormone replacement therapy, it will provide a simple solution to her problems with sleep.

Whatever the causes, lack of sleep leads to a number of outcomes that the patient would prefer to avoid. They include:

- fatigue during normal waking hours
- inability to concentrate
- irritability

- depression
- memory disturbances
- poor judgment

Physiologic changes that have been observed in people after extreme sleep deprivation also include decreased immune system function and poor wound healing (Doyle et al., 1993; McFarlane & Bashe, 1998).

SLEEP ASSESSMENT

An assessment of sleep problems begins with a clear history of past and present sleep patterns. The simple question "Do you have difficulty sleeping?" begins the assessment process and should be asked of all people with chronic illness. If it is not asked, many people will consider sleeplessness part of the disease, and not understand that it can be treated. Further, asking "Do you have trouble falling asleep?" and "Do you wake up in the middle of the night or early in the morning?" can help in determining the cause and potential treatments.

Symptomatology that interferes with the sleep–wake cycle is assessed by asking very direct questions. Some obvious but helpful approaches are:

Do you have pain that interferes with your sleep?

Can you identify anything that keeps you from sleeping, like noise or room temperature?

Are you frightened at night?

Treatment of sleeplessness related to symptoms requires treatment of the symptoms. Similarly, if the patient can identify a medication that seems to cause sleeplessness, the need for the medication must be balanced with the need for sleep. Medications that interfere with sleep include:

- stimulants
- bronchodilators
- some antihypertensives
- activating antidepressants

- diuretics given too close to bedtime

- rebound effect from withdrawal of sedatives, hypnotics, or analgesics

- long-term opiate use, though this is not an indication to withhold pain medication

- chemicals used in society (e.g., alcohol, caffeine, and nicotine)

After an initial assessment identifies the patient's perception of whether a sleep pattern disturbance exists, and the patient's identification of factors contributing to it, a more refined sleep assessment technique may be used. The use of a sleep diary documents the frequency and extent of the problem. A diary should document the sleep–wake cycle, including the sleep schedule, naps, activity, and medications used. The sleep diary should be kept for at least a week.

SLEEP HYGIENE

Sleep hygiene is composed of two things: creation of consistent patterns of sleep behavior and creation of a sleep-conducive environment. Consistent patterns of sleep behavior means going to bed at the same time each night; maintaining as active a schedule of activity in the daytime as possible; associating bed with sleep, and staying out of it when it is not time to sleep (as a patient's condition permits); for bedridden patients, providing stimulation during the day; and avoiding naps.

Creating a sleep-conducive environment means eliminating uncomfortable things from the sleeping area, such as ticking clocks, strong odors, or air conditioners or heaters that blow directly on an individual. In the hours just before sleep, avoid caffeine and alcohol. Give diuretics in the morning rather than at night. Provide blankets if required, dim lights if appropriate, and eliminate noise. Make sure the bed sheets are clean and smooth. Some people like a special snack, like hot chocolate, warm milk, or herbal tea. Although chocolate is sometimes considered to be a stimulant, if a person has been drinking it before sleep since childhood, the pattern is probably more important than the small amount of stimulant.

Sleep hygiene for the dying patient includes all of the preceding things and more. Nights are very long for people who are fearful and anxious. During the day, such anxieties are less bothersome because of distractions. At night, alone, the patient can be overwhelmed. The ability to talk with someone, psychotherapy if indicated, or the judicious use of medication may improve the ability to sleep. Medication for sleep can be counterproductive, however. As more medications are required for treatment of the illness or control of other symptoms, they may interact with drugs given to help a person sleep. When a person is weaned from the sleep medication, a rebound insomnia can occur. Medications for sleep should be given only for short periods of time, a week or two, while other therapies are tried. Pain and symptom control throughout the night are also necessary.

There are a variety of nonpharmacological treatments for insomnia that can be tried after the environment is sleep conducive and patterns of the sleep–wake cycle have been established. Behavioral treatments using standard progressive muscle relaxation, biofeedback to reduce muscle tension and stress, and brief psychotherapy to deal with fear are all helpful. Stimulus control (the sleeper removes himself from the bed if unable to fall asleep and does something else for a while), Therapeutic Touch, and massage also seem to help.

Movement

Regular exercise is a component of good health for everyone. People vary in their individual abilities to exercise, but the benefits of regular exercise are well-known. Positive results of such simple activity as frequent posture change have been demonstrated in circulatory, respiratory, muscular, digestive, and urological systems, as well as helping to improve a person's psychological state (Doyle et al., 1993).

For the person who is dying, physical activity can help lessen pain and stiff joints, increase strength in muscles, prolong a person's ability to care for herself, and improve self-esteem. It allows the person to continue in the family role for a longer time, maintaining an optimum level of functioning. It is a component of quality of life.

Many patients who have been told that the health care system has no more to offer, that there is nothing more that can be done to cure the disease, feel hopeless. They give up too soon, doing less than they are

The Game Warden

Mr. Gilliard, who was from a rural area in a southern state, lived his life for hunting and fishing. As a game warden for the state, he had spent most of his life outdoors. When he was diagnosed with colon cancer and discovered that the subsequent colon resection and colostomy was not curative, he believed he would no longer hunt or fish. He became depressed, with little reason to get out of bed each day. After discharge, hospice services were arranged. The hospice nurse learned that Mr. Gilliard's satisfactions in life were outside the house, and she helped the family plan to build a path from Mr. Gilliard's home to the river bank nearby. Once he had a reason to leave his bed, get dressed, and take care of himself, he spent several peaceful and happy months providing fish and crabs for his family. It was important to the quality of his life to remain mobile, to get to the bench on the river bank to feel the breeze, hear the crickets, and watch the sunset.

able, missing many hours, days, and weeks of pleasure. Careful assessment of functional status and an understanding of the things that make life pleasant for the individual will help the nurse establish a realistic plan for mobility to help extend the pleasure in life for the patient (see "The Game Warden"). Consultation with a physical therapist may be helpful as a part of the functional assessment.

MOBILITY ASSESSMENT

An assessment of a patient for the ability to be mobile can be incorporated into a general physical assessment. Pay specific attention to areas of weakness, especially knees and ankles. Identify areas of sensation loss because that means the body's normal warning system is not working. If feet or hands have lost sensation because of medications that change sensorium (e.g., due to some kinds of chemotherapy), they will need to be checked frequently for injury. Planned safety measures will be important, like careful reassessment of shoe size. The patient will need to avoid wearing shoes that are too tight because the shoes may become tighter (perhaps due to edema) without the patient noticing. Skin breakdown can become quite advanced before the patient is aware of the problem, and healing can be affected, perhaps slowed, due to medical treatment protocols. Include an assessment for balance and stability.

Check for dyspnea. Progressive exercise can be very helpful in improving respiratory function, but it needs to be done carefully with clear directions to the patient. Directions must include the physician's prescription for oxygen and medication use, pursed-lip breathing, and an assessment of stamina.

A patient was asked why he sat in the house so much of the time. He answered that he was afraid if he walked down the road, he would become short of breath and would not be able to get back. Fears like this are common and may be realistic. Therefore, plans to build strength and clear directions about how far is too far are important. Safety is a major consideration. It may be helpful to set progressive goals—walk to the fence on day one, to the end of the drive on day two, and so on. It may be necessary to walk with someone the first few times. A camp stool may be carried or a sturdy walker with wheels and a seat attached (available commercially) may be pushed while walking for balance and stability. A tired person can sit on it for rest periods. Once the patient feels stronger and learns to hear what the body is saying about fatigue, when to rest and when to go on, a regular pattern can be established. That pattern must be adjusted as strength fails. Pushing to meet a goal that is no longer possible is unsafe and can lead to falls and injury. Sensitivity to changes in physical condition is imperative, a part of competent nursing care that involves monitoring the patient and being present in the relationship.

RESOURCES

There are a number of devices that help people remain mobile longer. They include things to be carried, like walking sticks or canes; things to be pushed, like walkers or grocery carts; things to be grasped for support, like handrails or banisters; and things that can carry a person, like wheelchairs. Faith communities often maintain a closet or storage space for donated wheelchairs and other useful devices. This can be a useful resource. Recliners and comfortable chairs with footstools are helpful aids for people if they are constructed in such a way that people can get into and out of them without undo effort. Some patients qualify for Medicare-provided motorized recliners. They may have seats that push the patient up and out of the chair into a standing position. These are useful for avoiding stress in the knees. For example, one elderly man with pronounced emphysema and arthritis in both knees believes that he would be bedridden if he did not have a chair that helps him to stand. He can walk from the bed to a bathroom with a built-up toilet seat, and to his special chair. This lets him care for himself and spend time with the family in activities that they all enjoy. Without the special recliner, he would need assistance each time he wanted to get up.

When continuous bedrest becomes necessary, standard nursing techniques for position change and range of motion promote comfort. Because no one can accurately predict when a person will die, it is not appropriate to avoid turning a person, even if the turning is temporarily distressing, thinking that the patient will die soon anyway. Skin breakdown can occur in a matter of hours, compounding the discomfort. The same is true of stiffening, contracting joints.

Health care is an interdisciplinary effort (see Figure 4-2). Providers of care include not only medical doctors and nurses, but people like

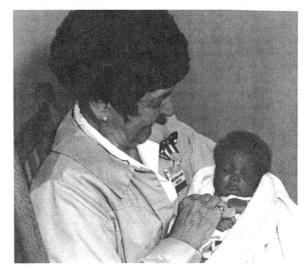

Figure 4-2
Volunteers rock infants, giving the message of comfort through touch. (Courtesy Volunteer Services, Medical University of South Carolina, Charleston, SC)

Mr. Bower's Back Rub

Mr. Bower was restless, warm, and clearly uncomfortable. He did not want any pain medication. It was not that kind of pain. He was just "achy." Ms. F. said, "How about an old-fashioned back rub?" He agreed. Ten minutes later his respirations were deeper and regular, his muscles were less rigid, and he was resting in the same position for several minutes. As Ms. F. withdrew from the room, Mr. Bower's comment was, "You always seem to know what to do to make me feel more comfortable." The back rub became a standard by which to measure comfort techniques. The question "Is it as good as a back rub?" became an evaluation technique. It also became a verbal reference to a shared comfort experience that reminded them both of the caring relationship that had been established.

physical therapists, chiropractors, social workers, and massage therapists. Each of these disciplines can provide care that improves mobility for some people. For example, a person who has back pain or stiffness of the hips may find massage of the muscles and an exercise program planned by a physical therapist of great benefit. Simple massage, including effleurage (deep or gentle stroking) and petrissage (kneading), can easily be taught to family members as a useful aid to care (see "Mr. Bower's Back Rub"). A chiropractor may provide an adjustment that makes it possible to become more mobile than the patient had been during the acute stages of an illness. Consultation with other health care providers, when that is the patient's choice, can be useful.

Touch

Touch is a basic human need. Without touch, an infant does not survive. Without touch, it is difficult to communicate love. Without touch, the elderly become withdrawn. And without touch, the dying person becomes isolated and depressed. Lack of touch is a form of sensory deprivation. Mr. Bower's back rub helped him for several reasons. The stimulation of the skin resulted in better capillary blood flow. Stimulation of nerve cells (sending rub messages rather than pain messages) blocked the perception of pain. He was also the recipient of ordinary touch.

Ordinary touch creates relationship. The skin contains millions of sensory nerve cells, and as such, is a giant organ of communication. It helps the caregiver assess potential problems. The first indication of a fever might be simply a feeling of warm skin. Cold hands, noticed during a handshake, might indicate anxiety or that a person has just come in from the cold. The skin communicates information. Touching is a way of receiving that message.

Messages are sent through the touch of the caregiver. The nurse can send a message of security to the ill adult who is walking with an unstable gait by holding the arm firmly, not gently. Holding the arm softly while applying a lotion conveys gentleness and empathy in other circumstances.

Touching is often incidental to the act of nursing. Touch may be related to performing a procedure (e.g., giving an injection); incidental, as when a patient is too close to another person and brushes against the arm of that individual; or purposive. Purposive touch can be planned to convey a message, assess information, or facilitate social interaction. All touch seems to have some influence on people. The nurse who practices presence in patient interactions will have an awareness of the kind of message being sent and will plan the interaction of touch for appropriate outcomes. For example, a back rub in a big city hospital during evening care might seldom get done because of the real constraints of time and other duties the nurse perceives as more important. For a dying patient, a back rub could have comfort outcomes that would make the back rub a treatment rating high priority. Touch might lead to less medication, less depression, and improved sleep and mobility status. The back rub for a person who responds to it in this way should remain a part of the plan of care and receive high priority.

Family members and friends can be encouraged to use touch as appropriate, so that the loved one knows the relationship is still there. Although physical intimacy may change as a person becomes sicker, the need for feeling loved does not lessen. Those who are fearful of hurting a dying patient usually are comfortable with holding hands, perhaps even applying lotion to them. In some cultures, the act of touching the dying conveys special meaning, so one's cultural beliefs must be respected.

Children should not be barred from a familiar lap if the patient is comfortable having them there. But if the patient's appearance has changed a great deal, a small child might be frightened and should not be forced to sit there. The message conveyed to the dying individual is not one of comfort in that case. The child may sit in another's lap, or alongside the patient and read a child's book to the family member, or tell of the day at preschool.

Caregivers should be encouraged to touch the patient appropriately, often, and with thought to the message the touch conveys: a warm, loving touch; a firm touch conveying strength and safety; or a gentle, "I won't leave you alone" kind of touch. In this case, intuition is to be trusted by those who have had a consistent and stable relationship with the dying patient.

Appropriate outcomes of touch for the dying patient who is experiencing discomfort include enhancement of verbal communication, facilitation of social interaction, and conveying emotion. The person who is dying is often socially isolated. Kolcaba (1992) identified four areas to address in meeting the comfort needs of dying patients. Ordinary touch meets physical, psychospiritual, and social needs, and influences environment. Touch affects every area of need.

In other eras, the dying person was hidden from view, shut off from the family or other people, and was seldom touched. A fear of touching dying people was common, and still is in some cultures. There may have been a good reason for that practice when the main cause of death was contagious disease. In fact, some HIV positive people believe that caregivers shrink back from touching them for the same reason—fear of contagion. There is no good reason for not touching the dying patient now, unless the patient chooses not to be touched for some reason.

Planned purposive touching requires careful assessment by the nurse. People learn the meaning of touch from families and culture. Hugging, for example, is expected by some as a comfort measure, but is an unwelcome intrusion to others. It is easy to ask a person, "Would you like a hug?" rather than hugging without asking. It can be uncomfortable and put up barriers to a relationship. A negative response can lead to a new question about what might help a person feel better, if not a hug. The answer might be something like, "Just sit with me for a while." The assessment prior to purposeful touch should include an honest appraisal of how comfortable the nurse is with touch, and what kinds of touch are acceptable. A sincere handshake is more likely to lead to a trusting relationship than an insincere pat on the back. For people who are clearly victims of social isolation, planning to include some sincere form of touch as often as possible is a valuable therapeutic act.

Nurses have developed or begun to use many therapeutic nursing treatments based on touch. They include:

- accupressure and Shiatzu
- Therapeutic Touch
- Reiki
- other forms of deep massage
- Traeger

Each of these treatments can be used for comfort, and each requires knowledge and practice to develop competency. They are described in detail in several places (Dossey, Keegan, & Guzzetta, 2000; Keegan, 1994). If not taught specifically in a program of nursing, the nurse wishing to add these comfort measures to an individual practice can get a number of books from most libraries; attend certified or approved continuing education programs, or review videotapes. Be sure you can document competence in the practice of these techniques, and follow established policies within the employment setting to assure safe patient care.

PHYSIOLOGY OF DEATH

No one really knows how soon death will occur for an individual, but there are some clues for caregivers and families to use to determine that death is very near.

A dying patient may be conscious to the end, able to communicate at least with the eyes. More commonly, a person who is close to death becomes progressively drowsier, waking less often, and then only to use a bedpan/urinal or take a sip of water. Communication becomes more subtle, and a caregiver may need to ask questions about what is wanted or needed, rather than waiting for a request for care. This change in conscious state may be more profound if the person is receiving significant amounts of pain medication. At this time, visits may be monitored so the patient sees who is wanted, but not so many visitors that comfort is denied. This, too, may be a cultural issue, and it is the patient who should give the clues as to whether visitors are comforting or distracting and upsetting.

Nutrition and hydration change during the dying process. When a person's mouth becomes dry and the skin looks dehydrated, it is tempting to try anything to relieve the dehydration. Chances are that one's nutritional state has been declining for some time. As the person becomes less and less able to take nourishment or drink fluids, caregivers need to consider what to do, if anything. There is strong evidence that starvation and dehydration are normal in the dying patient, and as the body slowly shuts down, lack of water and food actually ease suffering (McFarlane & Bashe, 1998; Callanan & Kelley, 1992). Forcing fluids and foods orally or in a nasogastric tube may add to nausea or vomiting or disrupt bowel action. Giving fluids intravenously may lead to pulmonary congestion and edema, even when given slowly. Giving only the amounts of food and water the patient is able to swallow is not the same as causing starvation or dehydration. The loss of the desire to eat or drink may well be the body's protective mechanism, an aid to comfort. Of course, a dry mouth should be cared for with premoistened swabs, sips of ice if tolerated, or a moist cloth. Lubricate the lips. Do not put a few drops of water in the mouth, hoping to relieve the dryness, or hoping the patient will swallow. The fluid is likely to be aspirated into the lungs. When the person is this close to death, many oral medications can be discontinued: stool softeners, vitamins, and the like. Others can be given in alternate ways, like suppositories for pain or nausea.

Most patients are unable to turn by themselves and require assistance. Involuntary twitches or cramps can occur. These quickly go away, and rarely is treatment needed. Sometimes a patient takes a last breath immediately after being turned for a linen change or comfort. If a family member or friend has been assisting, he may believe that something he did caused the death. This is not true, and the caregiver needs to be reassured of that fact.

Close to death the person's skin temperature may change. The temperature taken internally may rise, but the hands and feet become cool. Some changes in skin color may occur with the cooling, from pallor to bluish red with some mottling. Experienced hospice nurses recognize this as a sign of impending death.

Breathing is the change on which most caregivers focus. It becomes irregular, moving towards Cheyne-Stokes respirations: fast, then slowing, alternating with periods of apnea. If there is mucus in the mouth, as the air flows past it rattling can occur. Turning the patient on his side often helps this. Oxygen is indicated if respirations are labored. In peaceful death, respirations may become so quiet that when they cease altogether it takes a few minutes for those at the bedside to realize it.

These signs of impending death may occur together, or only one or two occur as a warning that death is near. The dying person often is able to look around one last time, perhaps have his face relax into a smile, and take a last breath. This is the time to say a last good-bye.

SUMMARY

Planning to keep dying people comfortable is critical to helping them live with a significant quality of life near the end of life. Comfort encompasses a spectrum of feelings beginning with a sense of relief from discomfort, and ranging to a feeling of transcendence. To promote comfort, it is the nurse's responsibility to assess symptoms that cause discomfort, and the patient's ability to function at an optimum level. It is difficult for the dying patient to maintain normal comfort behaviors, like getting enough sleep, exercising, and socializing, because of the declining physical and cognitive abilities associated with the disease processes. The patient's active involvement in making choices that promote comfort, combined with the nurse's knowledge and skills in providing care, increase the patient's opportunities to achieve comfort in her last days. A simple, gentle touch helps remind a dying person that she is not alone, and she hasn't died yet!

REFERENCES

Anonymous (1998). *Hospice care: A physicians guide.* Raleigh, NC: National Hospice Organization.

Brown, L. (1986). The experience of care: patient perspectives. *Topics in Clinical Nursing,* 8(2), 56–62.

Callanan, M., & Kelley, P. (1992). *Final Gifts.* New York: Poseidon Press.

Calman, K. C. (1984). Quality of life in cancer patients—an hypothesis. *Journal of Medical Ethics, 10,* 124–127.

Dossey, B. M., Keegan, L., Guzzetta, C. E. (2000). *Holistic nursing: A handbook for practice* (3rd ed.). Rockville, MD: Aspen Publishers, Inc.

Doyle, D., Hanks, G. W. C., & MacDonald, N. (Eds.) (1993). *Oxford textbook of palliative medicine.* Oxford: Oxford University Press.

Hines, D. R. (1987). *The concept development of presence in nursing science.* Unpublished manuscript, Texas Women's University, Denton, TX.

Hines, D. R. (1992). Presence: discovering the artistry in relating. *Journal of Holistic Nursing, 10*(4), 294–305.

Keegan, L. (1994). *The nurse as healer.* Albany, NY: Delmar.

Kolcaba, K. (1991). A taxonomic structure for the concept of comfort. *Image, 23,* 235–238.

Kolcaba, K. (1992). Holistic comfort: Operationalizing the construct as a nurse-sensitive outcome. *Advances in Nursing Science, 15,* 1–10.

McFarlane, R., & Bashe, P. (1998). *The complete bedside companion.* New York: Simon & Schuster.

McNeil, B. J., Weichselbaum, R., & Pauker, S. J. (1981). Speech and survival—trade offs between quality and quantity of life in laryngeal cancer. *New England Journal of Medicine, 305,* 982–987.

Nelson, E. C., Wasson, J. H., Johnson, D. J., & Hays, R. D. (1996). Dartmouth COOP Functional Health Assessment Charts: Brief Measures for Clinical Practice, Chap. 19 in Spilken, B. (ed). *Quality of life and pharmaeconomics in clinical trials.* Philadelphia: Lippincott-Raven.

Padilla, G. V., Grant, M. M., & Ferrell, B. (1992). Nursing research into quality of life. *Quality of Life Research, 1,* 341–348.

Pettigrew, J. (1988). *A phenomenological study of the nurse's presence with persons experiencing suffering.* Unpublished doctoral dissertation, Texas Women's University, Denton, TX.

The Dartmouth COOP Project (1994). Profile: Dartmouth COOP Charts. *Quality Measurement Systems, 1*(1), 25–39.

CHAPTER 5

Pain Management

THE PROBLEM

Despite the medical and health care advances of the last two decades that have made pain controllable for most people, pain has become a reality for many. Dozens of studies have demonstrated both effective pharmacologic and nonpharmacologic pain control methods. The education of patients and caregivers alike should focus on the fact that a person does not need to live in pain. Most pain can be controlled. Initiatives to educate people about pain control come from a variety of places, including grass roots movements and the federal government. The Joint Commission on Accreditation of Healthcare Organizations (JCAHO) has designed a new set of standards to ensure organizations look at pain as a coexisting condition, and treat it aggressively and effectively. These standards were implemented in 2001. Hospitals now consider pain assessment as "the fifth vital sign," to be measured on every patient at regular intervals, like blood pressure, temperature, pulse rate, and respiratory rate (Loeb & Passero, 2000; Patterson, 2000). Decreasing the fear of pain helps decrease the experience (perception) of pain.

Many older people believe that pain is a fact of life with advancing years. For example, when the doctor asked one senior citizen how long his foot had been hurting, the man said five days. "Why did you wait so long before coming to see me?" asked the doctor. The old man said, "I'm old. I'm supposed to hurt!" He had been walking on a broken foot for five days.

Cultural Perceptions of Pain

A nurse asked a woman in a bush hospital if she had pain. The woman had been out of surgery for about an hour and was fully alert. Her appendectomy had been uneventful. Every 20 minutes the nurse repeated her question, expecting that the woman would soon need some pain medication. But the woman became irritated with the nurse. She said, "I only hurt where the doctor cut me!" She could not understand why the nurse would keep asking such a foolish question. Of course she had incisional pain!

Part of the terror of dying for many people is the fear of a long and wakeful night full of pain. That fear is often well-founded. Two-thirds of the patients with advanced cancer, for example, experience significant levels of pain (Ferrell, Taylor, Grant, Fowler, & Corbisiero, 1993). The fear of pain reduces the perceived quality of life, influences the ability of a person to feel comfortable, and interferes with relationships.

PAIN DEFINED

One thing on which pain experts agree is that pain is what the patient says it is. Pain is a subjective experience, involving the total person. Pain hurts. Bresler (1979) said that pain is "a sensation, an emotion, a cognition, a motivation, and an energy." How individuals perceive pain depends upon many things, including education, ethnicity, culture, physical condition, experience, tolerance, severity, location, and secondary meaning.

Pain has meaning to individuals. A person who has had a serious accident involving a back injury may be relieved that pain is present, realizing that there is no spinal cord damage that would lead to permanent paralysis. Pain may be delivered by an abusive spouse, and mean fear and lack of love to the abused mate. Pain may be an expectation of changing life status, as in the old man with the broken foot. Or it may be something to warn of the need to take action. If the old man had been educated to use pain as a warning to take action, he probably would have seen the doctor earlier. Pain can be useful.

Dying people often see pain as deterioration in physical condition. Pain may or may not be related to a deteriorating condition. Abdominal pain in a dying patient may be related to the illness, or it may be a new problem that can be treated. Constipation, for example, is a common problem for people on multiple medications with little activity and poor appetite. Constipation can cause abdominal pain. If the health care provider believes that the complaint of abdominal pain for this person is a new stage in the disease progression, steps to relieve the constipation may be delayed and suffering experienced. All complaints of pain should be assessed adequately.

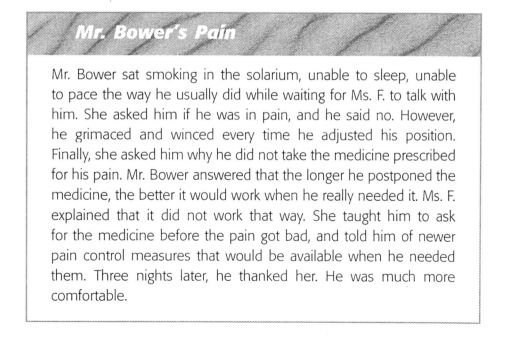

Mr. Bower's Pain

Mr. Bower sat smoking in the solarium, unable to sleep, unable to pace the way he usually did while waiting for Ms. F. to talk with him. She asked him if he was in pain, and he said no. However, he grimaced and winced every time he adjusted his position. Finally, she asked him why he did not take the medicine prescribed for his pain. Mr. Bower answered that the longer he postponed the medicine, the better it would work when he really needed it. Ms. F. explained that it did not work that way. She taught him to ask for the medicine before the pain got bad, and told him of newer pain control measures that would be available when he needed them. Three nights later, he thanked her. He was much more comfortable.

ASSESSMENT

Adequate and continuing assessment of pain requires three things. The first is recognition of the fact that a person perceives pain to be present. The second is documentation of pain treatment. Documentation of the progress/relief of the pain is the third. Many studies have shown that barriers to effective pain management include the fact that professional caregivers, including physicians and nurses, consistently underestimate pain and either underprescribe or inadequately medicate patients who need pain medication (American Pain Society, 1999). Patients do not report pain in a timely way, preferring to wait until it is severe for many reasons. The reasons may include culturally learned responses to pain; fear of becoming addicted; and not understanding when optimum pain control measures should be started. In addition, there is little attention given to nonpharmacologic treatments that have been shown to be effective in the relief of mild to moderate pain, or that potentiate the action of medication for all levels of pain. The first step in changing the inadequacy of pain management is to assess it realistically.

Professional caregivers are likely to rely on their own assessment of health status for most patient problems. Clinical decision making is taught in professional schools with an emphasis on objective evidence, with subjective reports often considered unimportant. The only reliable report of the existence of pain is subjective. Pain cannot be seen or objectively measured. The assessment of pain must be done first by the patient, and even unreliable historians or confused people should be believed about the presence and extent of their pain.

There are many good assessment tools that can be adapted to individual situations. Assessment tools are helpful in reminding caregivers what to assess regarding pain, and to keep an ongoing record of pain history, management, and treatment outcome.

Interview

The first kind of assessment that should be done is a structured interview in which the person with pain is asked to tell about her pain. After determining that the person perceives pain to be present, ask how it was managed previously, what kind of pain treatments help or do not help, and what kind of advice the person would give to a friend or family member in a similar situation (Ferrell et al., 1993). This kind of information gives the caregiver insight into how aggressively the patient is able to manage self-care. The acceptability and usefulness of different types of treatments are also identified in the interview. The patient can decide when to start a new course of treatment because the old one is not working. When the patient feels someone is listening to an important problem, it helps the relationship between nurse and patient and gives hope that the problem can be managed. Because most pain can be managed, that hope should be supported and encouraged.

The information from the structured interview can be recorded with more specific data on an initial pain assessment tool. This data includes location, intensity, degree of distress, quality of the pain (e.g., sharp pain or aches), when it started, and how long it usually lasts (McCaffrey & Beebe, 1989). The location of pain can easily be detected by asking the patient to mark a drawing of a person in the places where pain exists.

Rating Scales

Pain rating scales for pain intensity and pain distress are illustrated in Figure 5-1. In lieu of the pain rating scales presented, a person can be asked to rate pain using a number from 0–10, with zero indicating no pain, and 10 the worst possible pain. For some elderly patients, a Faces Pain Scale that depicts facial expressions on a scale of 0–6, smiles to crying, may be used (Flahaerty, 2000). These faces are elderly in shape, with wrinkled brow, different from the smiley faces a child's assessment form might use. Whether a written pain rating scale or the choice of a number to indicate intensity of pain is used, it should be consistently used with each patient, and written on a flow sheet so that the pattern of pain intensity can be traced over time. This allows the nurse to evaluate pain management strategies. The form is used to record regular assessments of pain intensity and treatments used for pain control, and has columns for other relevant information (Faries, Mills, Goldsmith, Phillips, & Orr, 1991). Figure 5-2 illustrates how a flow sheet to record pain intensity and treatment might be set up for Mrs. Foote.

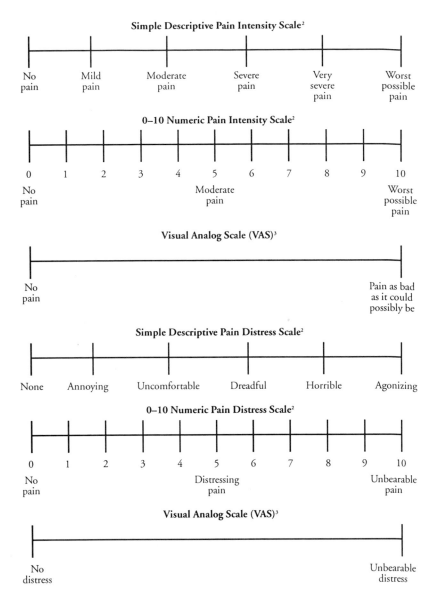

Figure 5-1 Comparison of Pain Intensity and Pain Scales[1]

[1]Acute Pain Management Guideline Panel. *Acute Pain Management: Operative or Medical Procedures and Trauma. Clinical Practice Guideline.* AHCPR Pub. No. 92-0032. Rockville, MD: Agency for Health Care Policy and Research, Public Health Service, U.S. Department of Health and Human Services. February 1992.

[2]If used as a graphic rating scale, a 10 cm baseline is recommended.

[3]A 10 cm baseline is recommended for VAS scale.

ASSESSMENT				MEDICINE	PCA		OTHER	
Date/ Time	Sed. Level	Resp. Rate	*Pain Rating	Analgesic: Drug/Dose/Route	Bolus; Shift	Shift Drug Total	**Nonpharm Therapies	Plan/ Signature

Sedation Level:
  0—Fully alert
  1—Relaxed, awake
  2—Drowsy, dozing
  3—Arousable sleep
  4—Unarousable

Figure 5-2 Flow Sheet, Pain Control

*Pain Rating: Use Scale of 0–10, 0 = no pain; 10 = severe pain.

**Nonpharm Therapies = heat, cold, relaxation techniques, imagery, and so on.

Adapted from Faries et al., 1991.

Mrs. Foote is a 43-year-old patient with cervical cancer who was admitted to the hospital to develop pain management strategies. She is in the late stages of her disease and is planning to return home to die if the pain can be controlled there. During the hospital visit, she will be taught the use of a patient-controlled analgesia device (PCA) using opiates, guided imagery to potentiate the action of the medications, and when to ask for changes in protocol. Professional staff will titrate the appropriate dosages of both the opiates and the nonsteroidal anti-inflammatory drugs (NSAIDs) based on her assessment of pain intensity. All of these things could be done at home, but her physician is also evaluating the need for further radiation treatments, and if the pain control is inadequate, anesthesia techniques for pain control. Because Mrs. Foote has determined that one of her important goals is to remain alert, the flow sheet has a column to assess her level of alertness during the evaluation process. Because respiratory distress and constipation are potential side effects of the opiates used, the flow sheet also has space to evaluate them.

The flow sheet used for her should be continued at home by home health, hospice, or family caregivers. She may be stable for a long period of time, but occasionally suffer from *breakthrough pain.* That is the term given to a transitory exacerbation of pain even though adequately controlled most of the time. Such pain is usually managed with additional medication, which may be needed for only a short period of time. Should a pattern of breakthrough pain be identified, she may want to learn cognitive strategies for dealing with the fear of such pain recurring. This is the time to use relaxation techniques (so that tense muscles do not increase painful stimuli) or imagery in which she could recall the feelings of security provided by a safe or peaceful place. Fear and peace do not coexist. Pain management protocols should be reevaluated if the breakthrough pain becomes a pattern.

The choice of a consistent method of rating pain intensity should be a policy decision of the institution or agency caring for patients in pain. That allows for adequate education of the staff concerning the meaning of pain intensity scales, resulting in more consistent pain management for the patients.

A Child's Pain

Children need a different way of assessing pain. Studies to learn the best way of measuring a child's pain are underway by a variety of researchers. Some use a poker chip strategy in which a child is given four red poker chips and taught to describe pain in terms of the number of chips, or "pieces of pain," experienced right now (Acute Pain Management Guideline Panel, 1992). Others use a series of simple faces, the first face smiling, the last one crying, and two or three in the middle in various states of unhappiness. The child is asked to point to the face that shows how the pain makes him feel right now. The child can be told if there is no hurt to point to the smiling face, if there is enough hurt to be a little unhappy to point to the next face, and so on. Once pain has been identified as present using this technique, the nurse can get even a small child to begin to talk about the hurt with such statements as, "Oh! You have a little hurt. Tell me about your little hurt. Point to your little hurt." The child can also be asked what the nurse should do to relieve the pain. Sometimes a hug is all that is required, but a big hurt will not be so easily treated. It is important to recognize that children do have pain, and it should be treated appropriately. Living with pain slows the healing process, causes distrust of the nurse and doctor, and diminishes quality of life for children, even as it does for adults.

THEORIES OF PAIN

By far the most common theory used to guide treatment of the patient in pain is the gate control theory. Knowledge of the physiological transmission of pain is the foundation on which the theory is built.

Transmission of Pain

Pain is transmitted from nociceptors, cells that respond to injury or painful stimuli. When nociceptors are injured, they release chemical substances that initiate the pain impulses and mediate pain responses.

Nocioceptors are located on the ends of neurons, nerve cells. Three types of neurons involved in the transmission of pain are sensory neurons, efferent or motor neurons, and connector neurons.

Peripheral nerve fibers are of different sizes, and conduct sensation differently. Sensory (afferent) impulses are conducted by the peripheral nerve fibers to the dorsal horn of the spinal cord. Chemicals, including neurotransmitters like acetylcholine, dopamine, epinephrine, and norepinephrine, help the impulse over the synapse (the space between ends of nerves). The impulse is conducted to the opposite side of the spinal cord, and travels along the spinothalamic tract to the higher centers in the brain. Some centers in the brain that are directly involved in perception of pain include the thalamus, hypothalamus, brain stem, and cortex. Within each of these areas there is a variety of functions, including memory, interpretation of signals, and emotional response. They are all involved in the transmission of pain (McGuire, 1998).

The gate control theory of pain proposes that a mechanism to inhibit painful sensory impulses exists within the spinal cord, in an area called the substantia gelatinosa. That mechanism is called a gate, and it can be closed to pain impulses by stimulating nerve fibers that carry other sensations, like touch or temperature. This is not an all or none phenomenon. In general, if many fibers of one kind are stimulated, fewer impulses get through using the other fibers. But the touch and temperature transmissions do not last long, and pain can quickly become the dominant impulse. In addition, the noxious stimuli can stimulate many more fibers that carry pain, and overwhelm the system so that touch and temperature do not get through. The theory explains why we can rub a sore area to make it feel better. We stimulate the touch sensory fibers and that decreases the pain for a short time. The usefulness of ice to numb a painful area is also partially explained by the gate control theory. The gate control theory is useful in suggesting several methods of pain control. Local anesthesia that stops the initial transmission of pain, or treatments that set up competition between fibers that carry pain and fibers that carry other messages in the nervous system (like ice and cold on a painful area or massage of a sore muscle) are explained in part by this theory.

Other ways of inhibiting pain use chemicals found in the nervous system. Endorphins are large polypeptides found in the pituitary and other places within the central nervous system (CNS) that prevent conduction of pain impulses within the CNS. They are naturally occurring substances with morphine-like qualities. Enkephalins are smaller neurotransmitters that close the pain gate by binding with opiate receptors in the dorsal horn of the spinal cord, thus preventing the transmission of the pain impulse. Chemicals (medications) of various types can be used to stop or change the perception of pain, both in the peripheral nervous system and in the CNS.

Research into the transmission of pain is increasing rapidly. The idea of multiple opioid receptor sites is growing in popularity. It proposes that there are specialized areas of cell membranes throughout the CNS, called receptors, that specifically bind with certain drugs or hormones (McGuire, 1998). Some researchers have proposed that these receptor sites increase in number, binding pain relief medications, if pain is allowed to go untreated or not treated adequately for some time. This suggests that pain should be treated in its early stages, not waiting until late in the pain process because that may stimulate the production of more receptor sites and make the pain more difficult to treat.

Perception of Pain

Because centers of memory, emotion, and learning are involved in the transmission of pain, they influence the perception of pain. For example, if a patient remembers that a particular kind of pain went away quickly in the past, there will be less emotion, less muscle tensing, and less fear than if the type of pain currently experienced reminds her of a prolonged, serious, and debilitating illness. If a person can focus, perhaps through guided imagery or another cognitive technique, on feeling safe and comfortable, pain may not intrude.

When pain becomes a severe problem for a dying patient, the use of a combination of treatments is advocated. There are many ways to close the gate to the transmission of pain. One way is seldom sufficient because there are so many fibers and so many components of the pain system that a single treatment aimed at one part of the system can be overwhelmed. A variety of treatments support each other.

PHARMACOLOGIC TREATMENT OF PAIN

Standards of pain control treatment suggest that moderate to severe pain usually requires some type of medication for adequate control. The huge variety of medication available, the multiplicity of administration techniques, and the potentially serious nature of side effects make decisions about the best method of pain control for an individual patient a difficult task for the health care provider. Although the primary physician or nurse practitioner generally is responsible for the order for medication, the patient, nurse, and family provide information on which to base the decision, and are often given the choice between doses and types of medications to be used within guidelines. It is very important that everyone who has a role in the management of a patient's pain be clear about the patient's goals and the principles of pharmacologic pain management.

The World Health Organization (1996) published a standard three-step analgesic ladder to guide practitioners in choosing doses and types of medications. Some kinds of pain, including that of low intensity, may respond to nonopioid drugs alone. Pain of greater severity requires a combination of low-dose opioid with the nonopioid. And severe pain may require higher-dose opioids with nonopioids. These basic principles apply to all age groups, including children.

Figure 5-3 synthesizes the fact that pain is mediated by two pathways, nociceptors and neuropathic, or CNS, involvement, and three steps of pharmacologic pain management. It should be noted that combinations of medications in different categories are often required and may be changed based on reassessment of pain levels. The American Pain Society distributes, at minimal cost, a comprehensive, frequently updated booklet that gives important information for caregivers on pharmacologic treatment of pain. It includes current treatment regimes, dosages, side effects, and warnings. It is a recommended reference for all those who care for people in pain (American Pain Society, 1999).

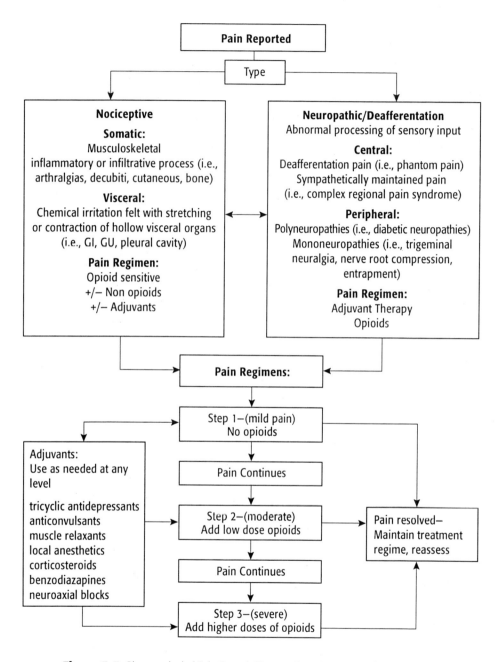

Figure 5-3 Pharmacological Pain Control *(Courtesy Betsy Bateman Rothey, RN, MSN, Pain Management Coordinator, Medical University Hospital, Charleston, SC)*

Patients who are dying may need treatment for acute pain when undergoing diagnostic procedures, recovering from surgery, or recovering from trauma or complications of disease, like fractures sustained during a fall. It is not reasonable to assume that because treatment is given for chronic pain, the same treatment will relieve acute pain. New pains need to be reassessed, and goals reevaluated.

Additives and Adjuvants

Some medications are commonly used to combat side effects of the pain or other medication. These medications may be added to the pain control protocols, and are sometimes called additives. They are different from adjuvant medications that potentiate the action of the main analgesic. Examples of adjuvant drugs include caffeine or tricyclic antidepressants, which are used to stimulate or change the depressive action of some opioids, making the opioid more effective. Phenergan is an example of a drug used by many nurses to potentiate the action of Demerol, although it is now thought to have no analgesia potentiating effects (McGuire, 1998). It can still be combined with Demerol to treat nausea and vomiting, and so is an additive.

Complications

Chronic pain is different from acute pain. The length of time the pain lasts, the progression of the disease process, and the development of some tolerance for medication require constant reassessment of the efficacy of the treatment being given. There are some principles to keep in mind when reassessing pain management strategies.

Less than one percent of people who take opiates for the relief of chronic pain become addicted to the medication (Ferrell, Eberts, McCaffery, & Grant, 1991). Addiction can be "defined as a pattern of compulsive drug use characterized by a continued craving for an opioid and the need to use the opioid for effects other than pain relief" (American Pain Society, 1999, p. 35). A physical dependency may develop after long-term use of an opioid, which is not the same thing as addiction. It can be managed with slow withdrawal of the drug, a scheduled weaning process.

This is aimed at avoiding symptoms like irritability, chills and hot flashes, salivation, rhinorrhea, nausea and vomiting, and others. Psychological addiction is uncommon in a population where opioids are given in sufficient doses to control pain until the pain is relieved, and then withdrawn according to standards to avoid physical symptoms. *Pain medication should not be withheld or given sparingly for people who have chronic pain because of an unfounded fear of addiction.* Patients who are addicted to narcotics or other pain medications before the problems with pain related to an illness begin may pose some difficult treatment decisions because the doses of medications required to adequately treat the pain will seem high. It is necessary to work with the person in pain to achieve the best possible pain relief. Everyone has the right to adequate pain control if it is possible.

One well-known complication of narcotics is the potential for respiratory depression. Some nurses are afraid to give the high dose of narcotics required to control pain because they believe that high doses of narcotics will compromise the patient's respiratory status. Research has shown, however, that respiratory depression is seldom a complication of narcotics administration if the patient has been requiring increasing amounts of the medication to control pain. It seems that the same mechanisms that lead to tolerance of the effects of the medication with regard to pain control also lead to tolerance with regard to respiratory depression. Of course, respiratory status must be monitored as it would be for all patients taking narcotics. Patients who are suddenly given high doses of opioids to control severe pain and have not yet built up a tolerance for the effects are more likely than others to experience respiratory depression. In that case, respiratory depression can often be treated effectively as a separate problem.

For the few people who do experience respiratory depression resulting from the only medication that relieves pain for them, giving the medication may pose an ethical dilemma. That dilemma is resolved by clarity of patient goals and organizational policy. If the patient's goal is to be comfortable, and the organization's policies permit it, the medication may be given. The patient and/or family should understand the consequences of giving the medication, including side effects. It should be clear that the medication is given for pain control, not to shorten life, though that may occur. If the patient's goal is for the longest life span possible, that person may choose to endure the pain rather than take the risk of dying. The nurse will continue to seek all available pain control treatments. A nurse who has a moral or ethical belief that makes it impossible to administer a medication for relieving pain when that medication may result in complications like respiratory depression will need to make other arrangements to help the patient achieve goals for a peaceful, pain-free death. A supervisor can help. Narcotics are not administered to shorten a life. That is euthanasia, which is illegal in most of the United States, although that issue is currently being challenged in the legal system.

Timing of Administration

Prevention of severe pain is more useful than treating it after it becomes severe. Consequently, it is important for members of the pain treatment team to understand that medication must be given before the pain becomes severe. Waiting until the pain recurs as an indicator of need for analgesia may be too late. Current pain control standards recommend the use of regular, around-the-clock administration of the medication. Monitoring the patient for the appropriate dosage includes the level of pain, vital signs, level of consciousness, related symptoms like nausea or confusion, and reporting the response of nonpharmacological pain control strategies.

A patient who has chronic, severe pain generally needs a medication that is released into the body continuously, rather than intermittently. This keeps the level of medication and the pain in balance, and the person can maintain a low pain (or pain-free) lifestyle. Recent technological developments have made this possible. Sustained-release oral medications and the transdermal patch are two examples. One goal of ongoing research in this field is to be able to offer a variety of medications that are continuously released to relieve pain more consistently.

Methods of Administration

ORAL

As a rule of thumb, oral administration of medications is preferred as the least invasive, easiest, and most cost-effective means of delivering medication. Some oral medications are available as controlled-release preparations. Morphine, for example, can be given orally in a controlled-release formula that reaches its peak action in 2 to 4 hours, but maintains a constant plasma level for about 12 hours. A twice-a-day regimen can keep patients who respond to oral morphine comfortable more easily than repeated injections or four hourly tablets. However, there are many reasons why moderate-to-severe chronic pain may not respond well to oral administration of pain medication. Some medications are not well-absorbed in the gastrointestinal tract. Some cause side effects like nausea and vomiting. Sometimes a sick patient has problems swallowing or digesting anything, including medications. When oral administration is not possible, there are many other routes of administration of pain medication.

RECTAL OR SUBLINGUAL

For medications that are absorbable in the G.I. tract, rectal or sublingual administration may be an option. These are usually temporary measures, and are dependent on the patient not having diarrhea, sores in the mouth, or other digestive tract disturbances that cause discomfort. If it is likely that the pain is not going away, but will become chronic, and the oral route is no longer available, a more dependable route that assures the same amount of absorption of the medication during each administration will be used.

TRANSDERMAL PATCH

One area of significant development is the transdermal patch. Fentanyl can be administered in this way. Transdermal patches are adhesive patches with medication in the center. They release medication through the skin continuously, as long as the patch is in place. This maintains a constant level of the medication to keep a person comfortable. Care of a person using a patch includes the assessment of the level of pain control, the maintenance of a pain flow sheet, and the administration of a rapidly absorbed pain medicine for breakthrough pain, should that occur. Skin care is important, and should be given according to directions that come with the patches. The old medication is usually removed, and the new patch placed in a different area.

INTRAVENOUS CONTINUOUS OPIOID INFUSION (ICOI)

Another method of continuous administration of medication (specifically opioids like morphine) is an infusion pump. The pump is set to deliver the medication continuously. An alarm should be used to warn of changes in rate of infusion or an empty chamber. When a patient is first started on ICOI, it is important to monitor vital signs and other parameters of safety every 15 minutes for two hours and until they are stable. Record the results on a flow sheet.

PATIENT-CONTROLLED ANALGESIA (PCA)

The patient is given a loading dose to achieve adequate analgesia before the PCA is initiated. Then, each time the patient pushes the button on the syringe pump mechanism of the PCA pump, a predetermined amount of medication is released intravenously. The medication may be in a cartridge-like reservoir located on a pump through which a regular I.V. is set up. Another option is a small, portable unit that can be attached to the wrist and easily carried around. The pump always has a series of safety devices to prevent accidental administration of medication, including a lockout mechanism that prevents a second dose from being given within 5 to 20 minutes of the previous dose. The PCA pump gives the patient the control in treating pain. The patient is encouraged to self-medicate via a patient-controlled analgesia pump before the pain becomes severe. Waiting does not diminish the need, and additional medication may be required if the pain gets out of control.

A nurse who is caring for a patient using any mechanical devices must be completely familiar with them, including how to set them up, safety mechanisms, potential dangers, and side effects of the medication. Standard care of the I.V. site is required, with special care for patients with poor venous access, to preserve the veins adequate for infusion purposes. Caring for patients who are on narcotics at home requires a thorough understanding of the narcotic laws of the state, and requirements for the documentation of drug use and waste disposal.

SPINAL ANESTHESIA AND NERVE BLOCKS

Epidural anesthesia is the infusion of an anesthetic agent, such as morphine, into the epidural space via a small catheter. Spinal anesthesia can also be given by using the subarachnoid space (intrathecal administration of medication). In both cases, the medication can be given by:

- single dose
- scheduled intermittent bolus
- intermittent patient-controlled epidural (PCEA)
- continuous infusion with opioid alone or with local anesthetic (American Pain Society, 1999)

An anesthesiologist inserts the catheter and administers the first dose of medication. In addition to monitoring the patient's pain and titrating the amounts of medication needed, the nurse has several other responsibilities when caring for a patient being medicated in these ways.

Complications of this method of pain control include the potential eroding of the epidural catheter into the subarachnoid space. This is likely to result in respiratory depression because of the larger dose of medication used in the epidural route infusing into the subarachnoid space, in effect causing an overdose. Infection at the insertion site and erosion of catheters into blood vessels are also potential complications. Special in-service instruction related to techniques of administration and potential complications of these forms of medication administration is required. Some policies call for apnea monitors, as well as frequent visual monitoring.

Nerve blocks interrupt the transmission of nervous impulses by injection of local anesthetic or neurolytic agent into or around a peripheral or sympathetic–parasympathetic nerve route. Local anesthetics are short term and easily reversible medications. Neurolytic agents are permanent, used as a chemical interruption in pain pathways. They are only done after careful explanation, trials with other forms of pain control, and for severe pain.

Most people recognize a local nerve block from a visit to the dentist. Dentists frequently use nerve blocks prior to potentially painful procedures. Nerve blocks for pain control can be done by local infiltration, or injection into nerves or ganglia. A sympathetic nerve block is done by injection of local anesthetic or neurolytic agent into the spinal cord.

Nerve blocks can cause allergic reactions, numbness and loss of both sensory and motor function, weakness of the part of the body affected, even hypotension. This form of pain control is usually used for a short time. If it is effective, a permanent interruption in the pain pathway may be made by surgical incision to provide long-term pain relief.

NONPHARMACOLOGIC TREATMENT OF PAIN

Surgical intervention, electrical stimulation, physical stimulation, acupuncture, Therapeutic Touch, and behavioral/cognitive techniques are all useful in the treatment of pain. They may be combined with pharmacologic methods of pain control, or in some cases used alone.

Surgical Intervention

Surgical intervention for pain control involves the interruption of nerve pathways in either the peripheral nerves, spinal cord, or brain. These techniques are not used for people who are expected to die very soon because the disruption in their lives caused by the surgery limits the usefulness. For the person with intractable pain, whose disease is expected to be in remission for a time, or for whom no other treatment has worked, surgery may be considered.

Acupuncture

Like surgery, acupuncture may be considered an invasive pain control method because it involves the use of thin needles inserted into specific acupuncture points in the body. These points occur along meridians, channels through which energy flows in the body, according to Chinese theory. The mechanism by which this occurs is not well-defined.

Although all practitioners do not agree about the mechanism of action of acupuncture (how it works), there is agreement that it does work for many people. It replaces chemical anesthesia for many people in China, and is used in pain control clinics around the world for chronic pain like that of arthritis and herpes zoster (shingles). Acupuncture has few side effects, and is economical and efficient. It may not be as popular in the United States as in Asia because of easier access to chemical products and drugs. Standardized dosages for drugs makes outcomes somewhat predictable. Acupuncture and other pain control measures that are noninvasive but related (like Shiatsu) are often dependent on the skill of the practitioner and individual differences among patients. Practitioners of acupuncture are now regulated in about half of the states. Names of acupuncturists who are certified nationally can be obtained through the National Commission for the Certification of Acupuncturists.

Noninvasive Pain Control

Margo McCaffrey, a nurse, is a major advocate and researcher in the field of pain control. She has developed several guidelines to use whenever noninvasive pain control techniques are a part of the nursing care plan. They include:

- Obtain a doctor's order for techniques not clearly within the scope of independent nursing practice.

- Educate all caregivers (health care team and family) about the purpose, frequency, and specific skills needed to implement the technique.

- Individualize the technique for the patient.

- Teach and have the patient practice techniques before they are needed.

- Start the technique for pain control before the pain begins or as soon as possible after it starts.

McCaffrey also emphasizes the use of the nurse–patient relationship in assessing the patient's acceptance of the planned techniques, willingness to learn and practice, and the general acceptability of the method (McCaffrey, 1979). Mrs. Foote, who was introduced earlier, was taught to use guided imagery for pain control because that was her choice. Other options might have included progressive relaxation or hypnosis.

Electrical Stimulation

Electrical stimulation is usually delivered by a portable device called a transcutaneous electrical nerve stimulator (TENS). It uses two to four electrode patches attached to a small, battery-operated box that delivers a mild electrical stimulation to the skin near the painful area. The patient can control the intensity, rate, and duration of the stimulation. The electrical stimulation is thought to work by stimulating the large nerve fibers, closing the gate of pain transmission. There are some preliminary data that suggest electrical stimulation might speed healing, especially of bone fractures. The mechanism for this is not clear and the studies are ongoing.

The patient who will use TENS for pain management needs to learn several skills, including skin care and care of the unit and batteries. TENS will be incorporated into the total plan of care. The electrodes should be applied near the site of the pain, but avoid any broken or reddened areas of skin, eyes, or the carotid sinuses. The use of hypoallergenic tape to avoid skin breakdown is suggested. While applying or removing the electrodes, the unit is in the off position. Once the electrodes are taped in place, the controls are increased in intensity until a mild, pleasant, local sensation is experienced. That sensation is sometimes described as tingling or buzzing, or even as gentle rain (McGuire, 1998). If it is uncomfortable or if muscle contractions are evident, the unit should be turned down.

Units vary, and the user should follow the manufacturer's instructions for care of the unit and controls. Batteries must be recharged on a regular schedule. Patients with other battery-operated devices, such as cardiac pacemakers and implantable cardiac defibrillators, are not candidates for TENS.

Obviously, the patient using TENS must be able to follow directions. As with other noninvasive pain management strategies, the TENS unit should be used before pain becomes severe.

Physical Stimulation

Physical stimulation techniques for pain control include application of heat and cold, and various forms of massage. Both heat and cold decrease pain by stimulating pain transmission fibers, and they both decrease muscle spasms. Heat tends to bring blood flow to an area, thereby increasing edema. Cold decreases blood flow to an area, decreasing edema and hemorrhage. Cold is also useful in decreasing itching, a common problem with people who are receiving many medications or who are in bed for long periods of time.

Mr. Bower's back rub (see Chapter 4) is the simplest example of effective massage. Using gentle stroking and kneading movements, the nurse stimulates peripheral nerves, limiting the use of those nerves for carrying pain messages. At the same time, the meaning of the act for Mr. Bower was that caring occurred, and that thought distracted him from the constancy of his discomfort.

Hand massage and foot massage are useful in accomplishing the same goals. The act of touching establishes connection with the patient. Foot and hand massage distract from the pain, and increase comfort. Some nurses practice reflexology, a technique of foot massage in which specific points on the foot are thought to correlate with different parts of the body. No physical connection has yet been established, but some patients report that reflexology makes them more relaxed and relieves their pain.

Shiatsu, a form of acupressure, is another specialized form of massage that may be useful in pain management. The practitioner uses the fingers, thumbs, and heels of the hand to press on the acupuncture points, rather than inserting needles (Dossey, Keegan, & Guzzetta, 2000). It is used in Japan primarily to maintain health rather than treat illness. It is a general pain management strategy rather than a specific technique for a specific pain. This technique requires special training.

Therapeutic Touch (TT)

This technique also requires some special training, and is useful for relaxation, decreasing anxiety, and pain management. Developed by a nurse (Delores Krieger, RN, PhD, of New York University), it has rapidly gained popularity in the last 15 years. Because it is based on the theory that people are fields of energy, Therapeutic Touch (TT) can be used as a nontouch technique without losing its effectiveness. This works because the toucher is working in the energy field that extends beyond the body. In the vignette about Judy, the use of the nontouch method of TT is described.

Judy

Judy was a 25-year-old woman who was admitted to the burn unit of a large hospital with burns over 95% of her body. She died six weeks later. During that time, she was subjected to the standard treatments for severe burns, including large amounts of fluid, hydrotherapy, dressing changes that were excruciatingly painful, and multiple medications. It was always considered likely that she would die. The constant pain required large amounts of pain medication. The medication was partially effective but left Judy with the inability to concentrate, confusion, and insomnia. She was very frightened. Asked if she would like to try Therapeutic Touch to help her be less anxious and possibly help with the pain, she agreed. The nurse followed the five steps of TT:

- centered herself
- assessed the energy field, looking for areas of imbalance or energy flow blockage
- "unruffled" the field
- modulated the energy
- grounded Judy

The TT treatments were done just before dressing changes, or before Judy wanted to go to sleep. She began to relax a little, and learned to practice breathing techniques to assist in relaxation so that she could control her ability to relax. Although the dressing changes continued to be painful, she was able to cooperate so they could be done efficiently. She was able to say good-bye to her loved ones and write her will. She died of infection.

There is an increasing body of research that documents the effectiveness of TT. Nurses are using it whenever anxiety interferes with a patient's ability to understand and make choices, as well as a part of pain management. When it is not a part of the basic nursing curriculum, it is taught as a continuing education offering or in workshops around the country. The practice of TT is dependent on one's ability to center. The practice of centering (a meditative awareness of self and the environment) helps and sometimes changes the nurse as much as it does the patient. Nurses report feeling calmer and less stressed after practicing TT, more satisfied with their ability to care for people. It is an example of two people (patient and nurse) in one energy field changed by conscious intention for the good of both people. As such, it is similar to the practice of healers from a variety of cultures, in which relationship is the core of healing. It is often taught to family members who wish to share this experience with a loved one.

Reiki and Healing Touch are two other energy field therapies used to comfort people, relieve pain, and promote relaxation. Both require special education by experienced practitioners and are taught as continuing education.

Behavioral/Cognitive Interventions

These interventions are useful for the patient who is willing and able to learn self-regulation techniques to help control pain. Visualization, imagery, and relaxation are effective tools for the patient to learn. They are useful in the control of mild to moderate pain, and to potentiate pain medications when pain is severe.

Progressive muscle relaxation (PMR) is the most widely recognized and used technique of this kind. The patient alternately tenses and relaxes parts of the body in order, either from toe to head or head to toe, focusing on the difference in the feeling of tenseness and relaxation. After some practice, the tensing part of the exercise can be omitted because the patient knows what relaxed muscles feel like. Fifteen to 20 minutes practice three times a day prepares the patient to use this technique before and after painful events (following procedures, after treatments like radiation or surgery, and so on). Teaching patients relaxation before they need to use it for pain control is important.

When teaching relaxation, a quiet environment and comfortable position in which the spine is supported in good alignment are helpful. Background noise should be kept to a minimum, or soft music of a kind that the patient enjoys may be used to distract attention from the noise. It is not necessary to cultivate a special type of speaking voice. A regular, medium-paced delivery of a scripted message is helpful. Three scripts for different types of relaxation are printed in the government guidelines for treatment of acute pain (Acute Pain Management Guideline Panel, 1992). Once the patient has learned the script, music can be delivered through headphones to block out noise. A relaxation script can also be delivered by audiocassette tape. This is a useful way of encouraging home practice.

Once a person has learned some form of relaxation, visualization or guided imagery is a logical next step. The nurse can be creative in developing pain management strategies using visualization as long as a few basic rules are followed. They include planning the script ahead of time, using images with which the patient is familiar, following the principles of physiology when creating images, and beginning sessions with relaxation. For specific pain management, images might include a peaceful scene. Peace is a feeling that is usually incompatible with pain. For example, one person with an injured, painful hand imagined himself on the bank of a stream with his hand dangling in the water. Words that included all the senses, like a cool feeling in the hand, green color and pine smell of the woods, babbling sounds and fresh taste of the spray of water from the stream, created a sensation of peace that distracted him from the pain. The feeling of coolness on the hand in the image may also have altered the perception of pain in the brain, helping to limit the noxious sensations. At the end of the visualization session, he told himself his hand would remain cool and almost numb. For two hours after the session, he remained almost pain-free, and was able to enjoy visiting with his family.

For people who have not been taught the use of visualization or relaxation preparatory to painful procedures or the onset of pain related to disease, it is still possible to achieve relaxation. Starting with simple breathing techniques, even a yawn, and using times while the pain is not severe for practice, the patient can learn to relax and imagine. If using PMR, it is probably wise to avoid the tensing phase if the patient is in pain. One way of initiating the process and achieving almost instant results for some people is to combine methods. Using TT to help the patient become relaxed, then leading an imagery exercise is a useful combination.

CREATIVE ARTS

The use of other forms of cognitive and behavioral therapies to help manage pain is limited only by one's creativity. Hospitals now have humor carts, which are described in Chapter 6. There are contests for funniest contributions to the carts. A good laugh provides a deep breath, distraction from the pain of the moment, and perhaps some endorphin release. The patient does not feel pain as deeply when laughing.

A loved pet, perhaps a cat curled up and purring next to a person in pain, is an essential part of that person's healing relationships. An old, loved hound who presents his head to be stroked helps a person recall times of joy, lessening the pain of the moment. For a person who is dying, the comfort, the touch of an animal may be as important as the touch of another person. The knowledge that the animal will be cared for after the owner's death is also vital to a sense of well-being.

Art is a useful tool in pain management. A child of six was asked to draw her pain. When it took the form of a fire, and the drawing included firefighters putting water on the blaze, the nurse suggested that ice might help the child's pain. The ice pack provided immediate relief for a time, and the child was delighted that the nurse had used "her idea." Adults sometimes use drawing in a symbolic way. It became routine for one man to draw his pain in an elaborate context, very dark, very structured, very detailed. He then cut it to shreds with scissors.

Humor, pets, art, and music therapy are all examples of creative avenues to explore for people dealing with pain. Most can be used within the context of a healing relationship, demonstrating a sense of care for the dying individual (see Figures 5-4 and 5-5). Sometimes they can be

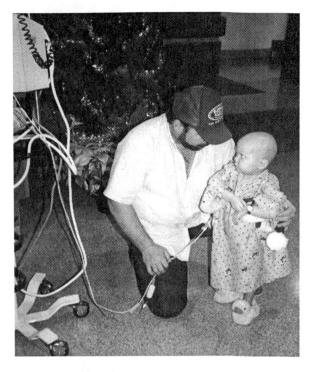

Figure 5-4
Children require treatment
in the context of a healing
relationship. *(Courtesy
Volunteer Services, Medical
University of South Carolina,
Charleston, SC)*

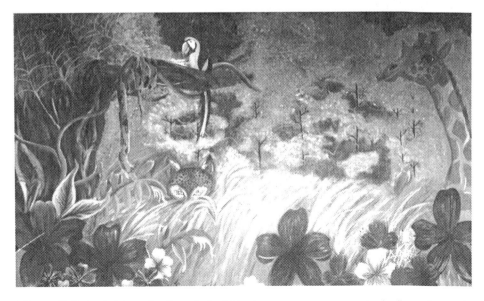

Figure 5-5 A colorful mural on the wall of a children's emergency room supports a healing environment.
(Courtesy Chris West, photographer, The Catalyst, Medical University of South Carolina, Charleston, SC)

used to assess pain, suggest management strategies, distract and change pain perception, and relieve anger. The relief of anger is important, in part because angry people so often tense muscles and move into rigid postures. Relieving the anger may relieve some tensing, which in turn relieves pain.

SUMMARY

Pain is a subjective experience. Many dying people will experience some degree of pain related to their disease process. They should know that it is not necessary to continue to live with pain. Most pain can be managed.

Pain has meaning to people. This chapter did not address the kind of pain that comes with loss, depression, or lack of meaning in life. But the physical pain that comes with disease contributes to those other kinds of pain, intensifying it and causing suffering. The combination of effective pain control and healing relationships helps to decrease that suffering.

REFERENCES

Acute Pain Management Guideline Panel. (1992). *Acute pain management: Operative or medical procedures and trauma. Clinical practice guideline.* (AHCPR Publication No. 92-0032). Rockville, MD: Agency for Health Care Policy and Research, Public Health Service, U.S. Department of Health and Human Services.

American Pain Society (1999). *Principles of analgesic use in the treatment of acute pain and cancer pain* (4th ed.). Glenwood, IL: Author.

Bresler, D. (1979). *Free yourself from pain.* New York: Simon & Schuster, Inc.

Dossey, B., Keegan, L., & Guzzetta, C. (2000). *Holistic nursing: A handbook for practice* (3rd ed.) Rockville, MD: Aspen Publishers, Inc.

Faries, J. E., Mills, D. S., Goldsmith, K. W., Phillips, K. D., & Orr, J. (1991). Systematic pain records and their impact on pain control. *Cancer Nursing, 14*(6), 306–313.

Ferrell, B., Eberts, M., McCaffery, M., & Grant, M. (1991). Clinical decision making and pain. *Cancer Nursing, 14*(6), 289–297.

Ferrell, B., Taylor, E., Grant, M., Fowler, M., & Corbisiero, R. (1993). Pain management at home: Struggle, comfort, and mission. *Cancer Nursing, 16*(3), 169–178.

Flahaerty, E. (2000). Assessing pain in older adults. *AACNNEWS, 17*(9), 5.

Loeb, J., & Pasero, C. (2000). JCAHO standards in long-term care. *American Journal of Nursing, 100*(5), 22–23.

McCaffrey, M. (1979). *Nursing management of the patient with pain* (2nd ed.). Philadelphia: JB Lippincott, Co.

McCaffrey, M., & Beebe, A. (1989). *Pain: Clinical manual for nursing practice.* St. Louis, MO: C.V. Mosby.

McGuire, L. (1998). Pain. In P. Beare & J. Meyers (Eds.), *Principles and practices of adult health nursing* (3rd ed.), 62–89. St. Louis, MO: C.V. Mosby.

Patterson, C. (2000). Shifting the pain management paradigm. *Advances For Nurses, Carolinas/Georgia, 2*(17), 20–21.

World Health Organization. (1996). Cancer pain relief (2nd ed.). *With a guide to opioid availability, cancer pain, relief and palliative care: Report of the WHO expert committee* (WHO Technical Report Series, No. 804). Geneva, Switzerland: WHO.

SPECIAL RESOURCES RELATED TO COMFORT AND PAIN MANAGEMENT

1. Internet resources on pain management:

www.halycon.com/iasp	International Association for the Study of Pain
www.ampainsoc.org	American Pain Society
mayday_pain@smtplink.oh.org	Mayday Pain Resource Center at the City of Hope (for education materials)
www.aacpi.org	American Alliance of Cancer Pain Initiatives
www.medsch.wisc.edu/pain/policy	Wisconsin Pain and Policy Studies Group (information on legislation and state policies on pain)
www.aspmn.org	American Society of Pain Management Nurses
www.painfoundation.org	American Pain Foundation (consumer information on legislative issues)
www.jcaho.or	Joint Commission on Accreditation of Healthcare Organizations

2. Addresses for specific information:

American Pain Society
4700 W. Lake Ave.
Glenview, Il, 60025-1485

National Commission for the Certification of Acupuncturists, Inc.
1424 16th St. NW, Suite 105
Washington, DC, 20036

3. Recommended pain text:

McCaffrey, M., & Pasero, C. (1999). *Pain Clinical Manual* (2nd ed.) St. Louis, MO: Mosby, Co.

Care of the Person
Who Is Frightened

THE PROBLEM

Anxiety accompanies many of life's changes. Approaching death is one of those changes. A common way of looking at anxiety is to consider it a general state of discomfort stimulated by new experiences. Fear is an anxiety that is more focused, less general. For example, a person is anxious about something going wrong, but fearful about an infiltrating I.V. Mrs. Nolan experienced a debilitating anxiety.

Mrs. Nolan

In the late 1960s, Mrs. Nolan visited her sick friend Mary every day until she died. The death was a hard one. Mary was in pain that was not well-controlled. Her room smelled bad, a foul smell that many believed to be characteristic of cancer. Mary cried a lot and could do nothing for herself, not even let go and die. It took a long time for her to die, although finally one night, she breathed her last breath. Mrs. Nolan believed it to be a blessing.

When Mrs. Nolan was diagnosed with cancer in the 1990s, memories of her friend flooded back, and she became so anxious she could not function. She knew that pain could be better managed than in Mary's time, but she feared many things: losing control of herself, of bladder and bowel function, of mobility, of the ability to think and to keep her emotions even. Her memories immobilized her so that she could not make a decision about her treatment, refused to see her family, stopped going to church, and began losing weight due to not eating. She could not sleep. At a time when she needed to practice good health habits she gave up exercise and began drinking alcohol to excess.

When a person approaches death, there are two areas of thought that dominate one's time and energy. One combines the apprehension of what is unknown with the desire to avoid what can yet be avoided (like pain). This apprehension is related to fear and anxiety. The other dominant area of thought is bereavement, the anticipatory grieving of the loss of this world and the people one loves (Saunders, 1984, p. 44). Past experience and present knowledge contribute to how a person resolves each of these issues. Grief and bereavement are discussed in Chapter 3.

FEAR

People who know they are dying experience a variety of emotions. They can move quickly from one emotion to another. A period of depression and withdrawal may be punctuated by periods of rage and anger. A serene acceptance of the impending death may swing quickly into anxious overactivity and a feeling of panic. Moods may last days and weeks, or minutes. A loving wife may yell at her dying husband, "Why don't you just die right now?" in her frustration of the moment. Any of these emotions in the dying person or the family and friends of that person may be exacerbated by fear. Fear is universal and normal, but not desirable.

Fear and anxiety related to death are sometimes seen in the physical status of the person. Fast heart rate, dry mouth, and quickened respirations are examples of physical cues that stress is overwhelming one's ability to cope. Insomnia and crying are also clues to identification of fear.

There are several specific fears that dying people frequently identify. They can be categorized as fears related to:

- symptoms and potential symptoms
- inability to cope and loss of control
- what comes after death
- changing roles
- loss of family and social relationships
- economics and status

There are also several specific fears that health care professionals who care for dying people can identify in themselves. Their fears interfere with communication. They include:

- the inability to do enough for patients (failure)
- fear of expressing emotions in front of others
- fear of blame for poor outcomes
- fear of their own death
- fear of eliciting an emotional reaction in the patient (Buckman, 1993)

Families who care for loved but dying family members experience the same fears as do health care professionals. An old man may not want to go into his wife's room when she is dying because he fears that seeing him weep might make it harder for her. He fears not being able to control his own grief as well as making her feel sad because of his grief. So, he denies himself time with her at the end of her life. He may also fear to take her home, not being practiced in the caregiving techniques he believes she needs. If home health care is an option in his community, the simple act of referral may help him to overcome this aspect of his fear.

ANXIETY

Anxiety is different from fear. A mild level of anxiety is useful in that it prods the individual to become alert, watchful, and motivated. A mildly anxious person takes in the information needed to make decisions and take action. But as a person moves from a mild to a moderate anxiety, the alertness changes to preoccupation and restlessness. It is harder to concentrate, and teaching is not as easily accepted. Other mood states, like anger, begin to intrude on the person's thoughts.

Common defense mechanisms like denial may push the anxiety out of mind, but it will reappear. Coping techniques other than defense mechanisms are determined in part by the coping strategies a person has used in the past, by culturally accepted strategies for dealing with death, and by the information and support the patient receives from the health care community and significant support systems.

If the anxiety becomes severe, the patient will experience physiological symptoms, such as tachycardia, increased blood pressure, dry mouth, diaphoresis, insomnia, and trembling. Pacing, irritability, fatigue, and deteriorating relationships are characteristic. The anxiety can progress to a feeling of panic. Mrs. Nolan illustrates what happens when a person approaches severe anxiety. In her case, alcohol abuse and withdrawal were attempts to put the anxiety out of her mind.

Goals of care for Mrs. Nolan and others like her are to use the state of mild anxiety to teach and support the patient, and to intervene appropriately in the stage of moderate anxiety to assist the patient to develop helpful coping strategies. It is important to prevent severe anxiety. Medication is sometimes useful for this, although there are a variety of other treatments that can also be useful.

COPING

Coping is a term describing the behavior one uses to respond to stress. Healthy coping is termed adaptive coping. Maladaptive coping is an unhealthy response to a stressor. Mrs. Nolan's use of alcohol as a behavior triggered by the extreme stress of a diagnosis of cancer and fear of death

TABLE 6-1	Behavioral Patterns of Coping
MALADAPTIVE COPING PATTERNS	**ADAPTIVE COPING PATTERNS**
Unconflicted adherence (same behaviors in spite of new information)	Traditional defense mechanisms
Unconflicted change (change in behavior because of advice of another, without self-assessment of the wisdom of the advice)	Vigilance, rational assessment, and action
Hypervigilance or panic	

Adapted from Janis, I., cited in Napholz, 1994, p. 43.

can be termed maladaptive coping. People develop a pattern for coping throughout life, and they tend to use that pattern (or coping strategy) for any stressor in life, including impending death. If the pattern is maladaptive, the individual may need help to change it.

Patterns of coping (see Table 6-1) may include the use of defense mechanisms defined by Freud. They are used primarily to avoid stress or conflict. For people who are unable to face a fear, especially the fear of death, denial is a defense mechanism that serves the purpose of protecting them from having to deal with the fearful situation. Although defense mechanisms are normal and often useful, if prolonged they can be harmful. In denial, for example, several kinds of actions may be delayed or prevented. They include a person's need to act in his own behalf, to take care of problems, and to sustain important relationships. If a person does not pay attention to these things, needed healing for patient and family may not occur.

Sometimes a person may choose to continue a familiar pattern of behavior in the face of new information that should modify the behavior. For example, people who are told that their disease is terminal, and there is nothing the doctors can do, may continue looking for the right doctor because their pattern for caring for self requires finding the person who can help. They are convinced that the right doctor can help. For an individual who is dying, this may be wasted effort, taking time from more important goals. It is maladaptive behavior.

Thinking clearly in the midst of anxiety, especially anxiety about death, is extremely difficult. Another way to cope is to take anyone's advice or suggestion without thinking it through. Mrs. Nolan might have heard a friend say, "Go have a drink and forget it," thus beginning her maladaptive slide.

A frantic search for answers may be another maladaptive coping behavior. Students who are not prepared for an examination often exhibit excessive anxiety, and try to cram for the exam—wildly searching for right answers instead of learning the information. Their efforts are generally not productive, so are maladaptive.

There are two things to work on to achieve adaptive coping. The first is to work on the relationship between the stressor (in this case, the fear of dying) and the individual. This requires increasing skills in perception (accurate assessment of the stressor and of an individual's strengths) as well as developing skills in intrapersonal and interpersonal communication.

A person who successfully copes with any problem or fear generally confronts the problem and seeks information about it. Problems and fears are discussed with friends and family or health care professionals (Clinch & Shipper, 1993, p. 61). Adaptive coping is seen in the pattern Janis (1982) termed vigilance. An individual follows a rational plan of action that includes assessment of the stressors (including sources of stress other than dying because a person usually has many stressors in life), a plan of action, and an evaluation of the effectiveness of that action. Mrs. Nolan will achieve vigilance if she can work through her denial, then consider the relative merits of her diagnosis (i.e., assess the real risk of death). She will decide what her resources are (including the people she can talk to), what the best treatments are for her under the circumstances, and evaluate that treatment as she goes through it.

This process is not easy, and almost never occurs alone. It is likely that Mrs. Nolan will be working through her problems, then suddenly become so angry at the unfairness of the situation that she wants to throw things. Expressing anger is a necessary part of working through the problem. Recognizing that, the nurse allows appropriate expressions of anger as well as expressions of sadness, loss, and all of the other emotions she may display. She may have times when she is unable to plan or to talk about her death. Later, she will continue the rational planning, and perhaps work on the relationships between herself and her fears.

The other part of coping is to learn to change some of the psycho-physiological results of stress for the individual (Napholz, 1994). Relaxation, humor, imagery, and biofeedback are some techniques people can use to counteract some effects of stress. People have learned to decrease blood pressure, tachycardia, and tachypnia, and increase peripheral blood flow using a variety of techniques. There is some evidence that some people can even improve the functioning of their immune system by using imagery, though not everyone agrees that there is enough evidence to state this as fact.

Not everyone chooses to try to learn to control physiology, especially if they are very ill. They should not be made to feel that they have failed if they cannot control blood pressure, or respiratory rate, or other bodily functions. Like other patterns of coping, the use of these techniques is determined in part by culture and experience. The competent nurse finds the healing methods that work for the patient according to the goals and values of that patient. For many Americans, medication is the treatment of choice.

ASSESSMENT

Ideally, adaptive coping begins with an accurate self-assessment of three things: the situation; the individual's own thoughts and fears related to death; and the other people involved. Individuals perceive situations differently and have fears that interfere with the ability to think clearly. An accurate assessment of the situation is often difficult unless a person can talk with someone who is able to reflect and clarify his perceptions. For example, Sam may become anxious because he believes he is gaining a great amount of weight from the treatments he is taking. After talking with a nurse to clarify his perception, he may decide to keep a record of his weight measured by a scale. This is a rational (logical) approach that will clarify the scope of the problem. Reflecting and clarifying what a patient is perceiving in relation to disease, treatment, and healing is often the task of the nurse. Setting goals, planning how to achieve them, and evaluating whether they have been met are mutual processes between the dying person and the nurse (or other caregiver). The nurse is often responsible for the accuracy of the information the patient uses to make choices. Examining a problem is difficult if it causes an individual to focus on it for long periods, and can lead to more anxiety. Mature coping requires accurate information to develop a plan for action and to determine end-of-life goals and relationships.

A sick person needs to know physical limits, and psychological and sociological strengths. Accurate assessment includes information about both the stressor and the person's coping skills. A person who has strong coping skills may function quite well in the presence of a very intense stressor, like the diagnosis of a terminal disease. Another person may need a lot of help coping with a small facial scar following the removal of a skin cancer if the coping skills are minimal.

Some stressors that require ongoing assessment for the person who is dying include:

- differences in expectations and goals between patient and family
- increasing communication problems between patient and family and caregivers
- problems in symptom management
- difficulty with anticipatory grief, low self-esteem, or early feelings of wanting to die
- guilt that one has done something to cause the terminal illness (Benoliel, 1991)

If any one of these areas is increasing in intensity, it may foster more fear and less ability to cope. It may take time and effort away from the accomplishment of important end-of-life goals.

COMMUNICATION

"Terminal care is a matter of human relationships . . . the challenge and reward of terminal care arise from the fact that it demands that we use the whole of ourselves to relate to fellow human beings who are in trouble" (Saunders, 1984, p. 62). It is most important to remember this when helping the dying patient who is frightened. There are differences in treating the anxiety of the dying patient and the patient who is anxious in response to other kinds of new experiences. For the anxious person, talking it out (ventilation) is the single most effective treatment. Yet, denial of death is common in American society, and this sometimes makes it hard for the dying patient to be able to talk about it. In addition, the family and other people important in the patient's life may be grieving, and find it difficult to talk about death. Helping a person talk about the immediacy of death in a personal way may be the most important care a health care professional can give. In the talking, healing relationships can be established, continued, or reestablished.

The healing relationship may have begun long before the patient was diagnosed with a life-threatening or life-ending disease, if there is an ongoing relationship with health care professionals—a family doctor, hospice nurses from a previous experience with the death of a loved one, a social worker, or a nurse on a special unit in the hospital. If not, a conscious effort to establish relationship should begin during the diagnosis phase of the illness. When the physician tells the patient and family of the prognosis, the nurse is usually present and stays with them to offer support after the physician leaves the room. If the family has questions, they can be answered quickly and factually as they arise. It is important to be sensitive to the family, establishing the rapport that will lead to a healing relationship. Ramona's case illustrates the help a nurse can give to a family in limiting the fear and severe anxiety experienced after hearing the news of a family member's impending death.

There are a number of useful communication techniques that can be used to develop a helpful relationship like the one between the nurse and Ramona and Julio. The nurse needs to take in all the information that is being offered by those in the relationship. The nurse needs to respond to them.

Ramona and Julio

Ramona entered the hospital for a diagnostic workup, basically feeling good, but with lymphadenopathy. Upon reflection, she remembered that she was more tired than usual, and her appetite was poor. After a series of tests, the doctor and nurse went to discuss Ramona's case with her and her husband, Julio.

Taking time to close the door of the room and sit, the doctor told them that the tests indicated a serious condition, a form of cancer for which there was little that medicine could do. He told them that there was always hope, and that about 10 percent of people with her condition did go into long-term remission. The doctor explained treatment options to a couple who was stunned. He told them he was available to answer questions, but that he would give them some time to think about what he had said. Then the doctor left the room.

Ramona began crying and Julio sat on the bed and held her tightly. The nurse closed the door and waited quietly. They realized she was still there when she handed them tissues. Julio began clenching his fists, and he asked the nurse how the doctor could be so sure of his diagnosis. Should they seek another doctor? For almost 30 minutes Ramona and Julio alternated their statements between "It can't be true—it can't be happening to us," and "There must be some mistake—the laboratory tests were wrong, the doctor doesn't know the latest." The nurse knew there was no answer to those questions, so she remained quiet, alert, and centered. Finally, Julio said, "Ramona can't die. I need her." The nurse said, "This is a time when it seems you need each other." She encouraged them to continue doing what they were doing, talking about how each of them felt and what to do about the future, together. She told them that they had some time, there was no rush. They could plan how best to tell family and friends and what information they needed to make decisions about treatments. She encouraged them to list the questions they had, and to include the hard things, like "Will I have pain?" She left with the promise to return in 30 minutes, sooner if they called.

Recognizing that each time she saw Ramona and Julio the interview would be different, the nurse reassessed the situation at each interview, never taking for granted their responses or their knowledge. She focused on helping them learn to confront the situation and get the information they needed to make decisions, and allowing them to discuss their fears and plans. Each contact, though different, was always characterized by the presence, caring, and competency of the nurse.

Taking In Information

Taking in information requires consciously attending to all that is going on at that moment. Paying attention is vital, the most important part of communication, and includes the use of self. The concept of presence, which was discussed earlier, is a part of paying attention. Honesty and a feeling of trust and respect are behaviors that help both people benefit by the interaction. During an interaction, it is necessary to control distractions as much as possible (e.g., by turning off a beeper or a distracting TV). It may not be possible to control all distractions, like the telephone, but fewer interruptions make it easier to pay attention.

There are some physical behaviors that help communication between people. There are very few times, if ever, that a health care professional should give sensitive, possibly devastating information to a patient or try to comfort a patient who has received such news while standing over the person. Standing while a patient is in bed or sitting, and trying to carry on an intense conversation can easily be intimidating and frightening. Some caregivers tend to link a soft voice with empathy. But if the patient cannot hear what is being said, trying to hear becomes a distraction that will not easily be tolerated.

The nurse should sit fairly close to the patient, facing him and leaning slightly toward him at eye level to see and be seen clearly. A summary of helpful behaviors follows.

- Maintain appropriate eye contact.

- Sit close enough to hear well and speak in a normal voice, but not so close that it is distressing for either person.

- Use an open, nondefensive posture to give an indication of the level of involvement.

- Avoid folded arms, rigid stance, or leaning backwards.

- Speak loud enough.

- Use all the senses, and notice if there is a change or difference, such as an odor, or if the person begins to feel cold and clammy. Attending to these sensations may help to validate what the patient is saying.

- Provide privacy and comfort during interviews and interactions.

Active listening is a total effort to grasp the facts and feelings expressed by others. The primary goal is to understand the situation as the other person sees it. Nurses are taught the basics of active listening early in their nursing careers, but emphasis on skill acquisition and information needed to begin a career sometimes means that the nurse gets little practice in really listening to the patient. Listening to the person is the major skill to be developed by the nurse, the area of greatest need for the person who is dying. Fear cannot be alleviated or symptoms controlled unless the patient is heard and the messages about the state of the symptoms or the effect of fear in a life can be assessed. A good active listener is:

- fully alert

- oriented to the here and now of the interaction

- interested in the person and what each individual has to say

- tuned in to both verbal and nonverbal communication

- able to suspend own frame of reference

- culturally competent

Responding

Taking in information during an interaction with a dying patient is only a part of the communication process. The other part is responding. Three basic but very useful techniques in responding are reflection, clarification, and silence.

Reflection is an accurate paraphrase of the essence of what a person has said. This technique lets the person feel heard and understood, and it does not evaluate the interaction. The paraphrase may include the facts or the feelings or both. For example, when the nurse found Julio in the hallway one evening some months after the initial diagnosis, he said, "My wife is dying. I'm too angry to go in there and see her. I'm tied up in knots inside, and she gets upset if I am upset." The nurse had three choices of responses. She could respond to the facts, the feelings, or both facts and feelings.

Responding to the facts, she might say, "You don't want your wife to see you upset." Responding to feelings, she might say, "You're angry." Responding to both facts and feelings, she might say, "You're angry, and don't want to get upset in front of your wife." Any of these responses are good. The best is probably the one that responds to both fact and feeling because the person will feel he has been heard, that he is not judged because of his anger, and he can continue talking.

Clarification develops, expands, and amplifies a person's comments. This is a useful technique when the person makes unclear or confusing statements. Clarification starts with a tentative opener like, "It appears that" or, "It sounds like" or "I think I hear you saying that." The nurse might clarify what Julio said by saying something like, "It sounds like you are saying that you feel concerned about your wife, but you think that her seeing your anger about the situation will only make her feel worse. You're afraid of what might happen to her because you are angry." This is helpful if Julio has not sorted out why he feels upset, and allows him to go on talking without being judged for feeling afraid or sounding unsure of himself. This answer also gives him the opportunity to correct any misperception on the part of the nurse.

Silence is a method of communication that allows two people to interact without the use of words. Silence does three things. It tells a person that it is not necessary to entertain the caregiver. The nurse will stay in the room even without conversation if appropriate. Secondly, silence allows both people in the interaction to collect their thoughts. It also encourages the person to continue talking after some time, without embarrassment at a behavior that might be less than appropriate in a social setting.

The rules of communication are guides, not rigid laws. Communicate a sense of wanting to be there. The act of being there, present, attentive, actively listening, and responding to need far outweighs any social mistake or slip of the tongue. The expert nurse caring for the dying patient is relaxed in the relationship, knows the goals of a healing relationship, and does not fear saying the wrong thing. The nurse is comfortable with silence and honest with feelings.

SUPPORT GROUPS

Though the nurse can help the patient with expression of feelings leading to improved coping skills, people who are dying are also very effective in establishing healing relationships with each other. Support groups are safe places for people to express feelings they fear others will not understand. The people who are undergoing similar experiences can offer each other understanding, the benefit of experience in practical matters, the knowledge that the group will remember them, and a safe place to be honest when families and others significant in their lives may be disturbed by their fears. In helping each other, each individual finds another meaning to life.

There are many kinds of support groups. Some are composed of people who are diagnosed with an incurable disease at the same time. More often, a particular institution or group like hospice has one or more support groups available to those who wish to take advantage of them. Some groups are composed of patient and spouse, some include children, some are only for the individual patients. Most groups meet for 45 minutes to an hour, but some groups meet for retreats of a weekend or even a week. Some are focused on specific problems, like anticipatory bereavement. Others are open to any topic. Some have leaders who are

Mary Ann and Roger

Roger needed a heart transplant. His cardiac disease was progressing slowly, his cardiac output decreasing and his fatigue level increasing. It was unlikely he would get a heart in time. A well-qualified clinical nurse specialist had started a support group for people like Roger and his wife. Beginning with an invitation to those people whose names are on the transplant list, the nurse scheduled a time and place in the heart center to meet, and parking vouchers for group members coming to a meeting. Both Roger and Mary Ann were invited. In the 12 weeks that Mary Ann and Roger were a part of the group, they were able to share their constant uncertainty mixed with hope, and their frustrations when Roger's condition began deteriorating significantly and it became clear he would die soon.

When Mary Ann returned to the group after the funeral to say good-bye to the people who had shared such a significant part of her life, they held a brief ceremony to commemorate his life, a kind of healing service. Special things Roger had shared in the group were remembered, and written messages were collected and burned in a small dish, the smoke carrying the messages upward to him. This physical act was a symbolic method of saying good-bye, but Mary Ann was comforted in the knowledge that Roger would be remembered by this group of people.

professional health care providers. Others are led by the members. Some are even meant to carry on after a person has died, to support the spouse or loved ones.

Camp Bluebird is an example of a special support group for adults with cancer. Not all of those who attend this weekend retreat will die of the disease, but many will. They spend the weekend in a beautiful, natural setting, with individual rooms at a lodge, in the company of each other and volunteers who teach a variety of skills. Some volunteers focus on comfort techniques, allowing the campers to experience massage,

Therapeutic Touch, imagery, and meditation. Others focus on self-esteem techniques, like makeovers, choice of wigs, and color and style hints for buying new clothes. Connections with loved ones who are not present are maintained by asking significant people in the campers' lives ahead of time to send a special letter, telling the camper something special about their relationship. The letters are shared as the campers wish, during a time that tends to be quite emotional. Each member of the group builds a bird house, which symbolizes hope. There are several group meetings for ventilation, sharing, and support. Campers return to family, friends, home, or care setting feeling refreshed, renewed, and hopeful. Some of them report a kind of transcendent or spiritual experience.

When starting a support group, several things must be considered (Anonymous, 1999). It is helpful to a novice to have the assistance of someone experienced in leading support groups. Competency involves an understanding of group process, the ability to make a clear choice about leadership style (e.g., directive versus nondirective), an unambiguous statement about the purpose of the group, the establishment of membership criteria for the group, and adherence to accountability standards for support groups. Accountability standards assure that the group is a place for safe disclosure.

- Information shared in the group is confidential.
- Members of the group are anonymous outside the group.
- Each person in the group is heard and respected.
- Limitations of the group are acknowledged. That is, psychotherapy is not done in a support group unless a highly qualified professional leader has convened the group and established that as its purpose.

The group should also have some structure. Prior to the first session, those who form the group should have decided:

- purpose and goals
- group size
- location

- length of sessions
- group roles
- frequency of meetings
- resources available
- when the group should disband (Adapted from LaSalle & LaSalle, 1998).

For a group of people who may be dying, some understanding by the group leader of the problems the group members are experiencing may be helpful. For example, if the common problem is increasing loss of control, as in multiple sclerosis, the group will probably share feelings of chronic anxiety more than acute anxiety. The need for specific kinds of information is different in that group from a group waiting for transplants. If the group's purpose is to share feelings rather than get information, the ability to interpret care and treatment plans is less important.

Common needs often addressed in a support group include:

- obtaining guidance
- reassurance of worth
- a sense of reliable alliance among members
- opportunities for nurturance
- attachment
- social integration (adapted from Kinney, Mannetter, & Carpenter, 1985)

Meeting this set of needs gives the group members additional resources to use in coping with fear and anxiety.

OTHER TECHNIQUES FOR REDUCTION OF FEAR AND ANXIETY

There are several other nursing interventions useful in helping a person control fear and anxiety related to dying. Visualization, humor, and life review are three of these techniques.

Visualization

Visualization, seeing something with the mind's eye or making a mental image of something, is a technique often suggested for stress control and healing (Keegan, 1994). Based on the idea that the mind and body are so interconnected that a change in one corresponds in general to a change in the other, people use visualization or specific imagery to decrease feelings of distress. If a person can imagine a scene that makes him feel peaceful, the whole body begins to relax and the signs of anxiety diminish. Anxiety cannot coexist with relaxation.

Everyone has had the experience of imagination. It is a universal human phenomenon. People imagine what it is like to receive an award, meet a great person, or win a special competition. Imagining the tart taste of a lemon or the sweetness of cold ice cream makes the mouth water.

Using this natural ability, a person can create a place in the mind that is unique. The created place can contain all the things believed to be necessary for comfort or peace. It is always available and always safe. A skillful nurse can guide the patient in the creation of this place so that it is useful for dealing with the fear related to dying.

When a nurse or someone else guides the creation of an image, the process is termed guided imagery. There are many forms of imagery. The safe-place technique is a process image, an image that can continually be changed as needs change. In guiding the creation of such an image, the nurse builds on several ideas.

- A relaxation exercise is a useful first step when teaching a patient to create the safe place.

- The safe place should be a place that appears soon into the exercise. Do not spend time looking for an ideal image to appear.

- A person can imagine getting to the safe place in a variety of ways, such as taking an elevator up (or down), being carried away by a cloud, or being blown by the wind.

- Indirect suggestions allow the patient to be creative and choose the most comfortable images.

- Daily practice in visiting the safe place helps make it more accessible during particularly stressful times.

- There should be a planned method of reentering the world outside the safe place or image; for example, reversing the steps taken to get into the safe place or exiting the safe place via a slide or another appropriate image.

Mrs. Pond

One dying patient, Mrs. Pond, experienced nightmares involving dying with no one present. She woke up nights in a cold sweat, calling out to her husband and children to hold her hand and stay with her. Before the onset of the nightmares, she had learned to use progressive muscle relaxation for pain control. The nurse suggested she build on that relaxation technique and create a safe place image to help with the anxiety that came after the nightmares. The nurse helped her with a regular progressive relaxation session, and toward the end of it made the indirect suggestion that Mrs. Pond find herself transported across time and space to a place that meant peace and happiness. After a short time of silence, further suggestions were made that Mrs. Pond notice everything in the safe place and remember it so she could return to it later, and that she be transported back to the present feeling refreshed and calm.

Mrs. Pond later reported that during the session she found herself on a sled, being whisked through the air like Santa Claus to a place filled with light, warmth, and soft animals—rabbits, koala bears, and most importantly, a large white cat. The cat immediately curled up on her lap, purring and offering the comfort only animals can give, in this case a very tactile kind of support. The nurse reminded Mrs. Pond that she could return to her safe place during any relaxation session, even after an upsetting nightmare, and recapture the feeling of peace and of being loved. She needed only to become relaxed and call her sled.

Imagery can also be used to rehearse an event about which a person is fearful. It is well-known that prior to chemotherapy some patients become nauseated and even vomit in anticipation of the treatment, almost living the event before it happens. Rehearsing the session of chemotherapy as imagery allows the patient to create more positive outcomes in the images; for example, a session in which no vomiting occurs. The body will often respond to the rehearsed sensations as practiced.

The imagery used to rehearse a situation (surgery, endoscopic examination, medication, and so on) should be based on accurate information. If the procedure is uncomfortable, that fact should be included. It can be related to something coped with successfully in the past, and be given positive meaning. For example, a procedure requiring a needle insertion may be related to a past mosquito bite, with the suggestion that the patient has successfully managed bites before. If a medication burns while being infused into a vein, the image can be one of power and strength of medication being sent to fight disease. Power surging through the body can be transformed into energy, the ability to eat or take fluids, or whatever is realistic in the situation—the positive goal set by patient and nurse together.

It is also possible for the patient to imagine what it feels like to die. Suggesting this to a relaxed patient should only be done by someone experienced in caring for dying patients. It is a useful technique for helping a person cope with the reality of dying, but the caregiver must be able to handle the needs the patient brings up as a result of the session.

Guided imagery is a planned intervention, and it takes some skill to use it effectively. It is not used to run away from problems or avoid dealing with issues. The patient is still given all the information needed to make decisions, and time to talk about problems. Social interactions are still vital. The image of a safe place gives a kind of time out from the intensity of a situation, and can refresh and strengthen a patient so that issues can be addressed calmly.

Humor

Laughter and humor make a person feel good. Even scripture says "a merry heart doeth good like a medicine . . ." (Proverbs 17:22). Humor helps promote health physically, as in the respiratory effects of a deep laugh; psychologically, as a coping skill; and cognitively, as a distraction (Sherman, 2000). It can turn a negative event into a less intense one. There are few negative effects of humor, though a patient must be made to feel that people are laughing with him, not at him, or a sense of distrust will develop.

The appropriate use of humor begins with caregivers who are able to have fun together. In a creative and open environment, nurses who are able to laugh at themselves and with others are able to communicate more freely and experience less tension in the work setting (Wooten, 1996). That freedom allows the caregiver to laugh at the jokes the patient tells, and in turn, the shared laughter brings the two closer together in the healing relationship.

Other uses of humor include:

- ice breaker
- decrease stress
- cope with emotions
- release anger
- facilitate learning
- promote socialization
- manage a delicate situation
- share vulnerability
- improve communication
- release hostility
- provide distraction
- give reassurance

The ability to tell a funny story may not be everyone's talent. But everyone can laugh, appreciate a good story, and perceive things in the situation as funny, odd, or ironic. Many people can contribute to the development and use of a humor cart, box, or bag. Used in places where patients may have to stay a long time, the humor cart can be a planned

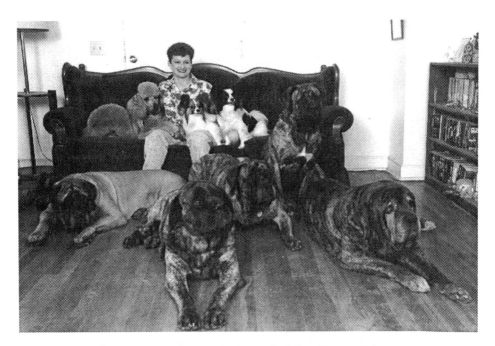

Figure 6-1 Pet therapy animals come in all sizes. *(Courtesy Volunteer Services, Medical University of South Carolina, Charleston, SC)*

nursing intervention for anyone who needs a good laugh. Some items that might be included are funny videotapes, joke books, cartoons, disguise kits, clown noses, hats, rubber spiders, whoopee cushions, plastic food or drink, and anything else people contribute that makes them laugh. Pet therapy animals help people laugh (see Figure 6-1).

Humor can also indicate that a person is beginning to recover from a tense, stress-filled event. Two brothers and a father stopped in a restaurant after the funeral of a third brother. They had been through an intense confrontation with death and had found support in each other. They had a short time until they would separate and go to their own homes. When the server asked for the predinner drink orders, the responses were: martini-dry; martini-very dry; cola-wet. The server laughed at the "wet," the family began to laugh, and each knew at that moment that the others would be all right and would get through the grief. The joke was small, but the meaning was significant.

Life Review

Life review is a nursing intervention in which a person is led through a remembrance of life, stage by stage. It is a kind of reminiscence that is structured and planned. Life review has been shown to help prevent depression, and help depressed people and people dealing with end-of-life issues to work toward a sense of integration of life events, a sense that their lives are unique and meaningful (Haight, 1991; Haight, Michel, & Hendrix, 1998). When a person at the end of life is anxious due to a sense of meaninglessness and alienation, planned life review may help.

People who have lived through a near-death experience (NDE) often report that during the experience they saw every event in their lives in exactly the same moment. Graduations, weddings, funerals, and every other important event occurred at the same time during the NDE. Interestingly, old people, who tend to reminisce naturally and without help, do not report life review as a part of the NDEs they may have. Some researchers believe that this is evidence for the fact that the life review is such an important psychological task that if a person does not do it beforehand, the person will do it at the moment of death.

Life review can be conducted in a group, but it is more effective individually. The six to eight sessions parallel Erickson's stages of life, from birth to old age, beginning with the first memory. Open-ended questions for each session/stage can be guided by Haight's Life Review and Experiencing Form (LREF) (see Appendix 1). Each session is about 45 minutes in length. As a person goes through the work of reviewing life events honestly, pain may be felt because part of life has been painful. But toward the end of the sessions, and particularly in a summary session, an individual usually begins to feel a sense of integration with the past and the present, a kind of wholeness to life. This leads, in turn, to greater peace, less unfinished business, and transcendence.

When conducting life review for young people who are dying, not all the stages will be represented. But a life, no matter how long, is still a complete life. Assisting a patient to see life as a whole is part of the healing process.

Conducting Life Review sessions with individuals is a skill. As such, it can be learned and become a useful tool for nurses, social workers, and other health care professionals. It requires:

- learning the process
- time and environment for sessions
- excellent communication and interview skills
- ability to deal with potentially difficult memories and unresolved problems

Those who choose not to learn the formal skill of Life Review should still value the process and the need for reminiscence. Allow people to share memories, even if they share the same ones many times. It is an important part of the process of understanding one's meaning in life.

PSYCHIATRIC ILLNESS IN DYING

Although fear and anxiety are common problems for those who are dying, and can often be helped using the techniques and nursing treatments discussed previously, psychiatric disorders are different and require different treatment. Psychiatric disorders may be a problem for some dying people before they acquire the terminal disease, and the fact that they are dying does not alter that. Psychiatric illness may also be stimulated by the illness. Anxiety may become panic, a person in pain may become depressed, a dementia may develop as a result of an organic process found in HIV infection or a brain metastasis. All of these conditions are treatable.

Treatment of psychiatric conditions is necessary to achieve the goal of care for people who are dying: to be alert and aware, able to communicate with loved ones, with symptoms controlled until the time of death. Another reason for starting or continuing psychiatric treatment for people who need it is that the illness may make it difficult to care for them if they are not treated. For example, a person may become hostile and combative because of paranoia associated with organic brain disease. Treatment of the psychiatric problem requires special expertise, and if successful, makes the healing relationship much easier to achieve.

Panic, depression, and dementias are conditions that the nurse should not deal with alone. Because they often require medication and/or psychotherapy, referral to a qualified team member is an appropriate option. If untreated, patients are at risk for insomnia, attempts at suicide, and the inability to form or continue supportive, healing relationships. Resources for psychiatric referrals are listed in Table 6-2.

TABLE 6-2   Resources for Treatment of Psychiatric Illness in Dying Patients

Advanced practice nurses:*
Psychiatric nurse practitioners
Clinical nurse specialists in psychiatric nursing
Psychiatric liaison nurses

Psychiatrists and some medical doctors

Emergency psychiatric services:
Mobile crisis units
Psychiatric liaison teams in hospitals
Hot lines offering referral services for special symptoms, such as threats of suicide

Psychiatric counselors, depending on licensing laws in each state:
Psychologists
Social workers

*Some advanced practice nurses have prescriptive privileges, and can offer both counseling and medication.

SUMMARY

People who are dying often fear the night, the process of death, losing loved ones, and pain and suffering. They may become increasingly anxious. Using excellent communication skills, the nurse helps the individual and family to develop coping skills, and works toward developing a healing relationship. Within the healing relationship, patient, family, and nurse have choices about appropriate techniques to use to decrease fear and anxiety, such as support groups, visualization, humor, or life review. The nurse who establishes a healing relationship with a fearful or anxious patient helps that person to live more fully until death occurs.

REFERENCES

Anonymous (1999). For maximum effectiveness, carefully design structure for support group: Provide consistent evaluation to determine if outcomes are achieved. *Patient Education Management, 6*(3), 25–27.

Benoliel, J. (1991). Multiple meanings of death for older persons. In E. M. Baines (Ed.), *Perspectives on gerontological nursing,* Newbury Park, CA: Sage Publications.

Buckman, R. (1993). Communication in palliative care: A practical guide. In D. Doyle, G. W. C. Hanks, & N. MacDonald (Eds.), *Oxford textbook of palliative medicine.* Oxford: Oxford University Press.

Clinch, J., & Shipper, H. (1993). Quality of life assessment in palliative care. In D. Doyle, G. W. C. Hanks, & N. MacDonald (Eds.), *Oxford textbook of palliative medicine.* Oxford: Oxford University Press.

Haight, B. K. (1991). Psychological illness in aging. In E. M. Baines (Ed.), *Perspectives on gerontological nursing.* Newbury Park, CA: Sage Publications.

Haight, B. K., Michel, Y., & Hendrix, S. (1998). Life review: Preventing despair in newly relocated nursing home residents, short- and long-term effects. *The International Journal of Aging and Human Development, 47*(2), 119–142.

Janis, I. (1982). *Stress, attitudes and decisions: Selected papers.* New York: Praeger Publishers.

Keegan, L. (1994). *The nurse as healer.* Albany, NY: Delmar.

Kinney, C. K. D., Mannetter, R., & Carpenter, M. (1985). Support groups. In G. M. Bulachek & J. C. McCloskey (Eds.), *Nursing interventions: Treatments for nursing diagnoses.* Philadelphia: W.B. Saunders Co.

LaSalle, P., & LaSalle, A. (2001). Therapeutic groups. In G. Stuart & M. Laraia (Eds.), *Principles and Practices of Psychiatric Nursing* (7th ed.) St. Louis, MO: Mosby, Inc.

Napholz, L. (1994). Promoting adaptive responses to stressors. In P. Beare & J. Myers (Eds.), *Principles and practices of adult health nursing.* St. Louis, MO: C.V. Mosby Co.

Saunders, C. (1984). *The management of terminal malignant disease* (2nd ed.). London: Edward Arnold Publishers, Ltd.

Sherman, K. M. (2000). Therapeutic humor: A coping tool for cancer patients and nurses. *Holistic Nursing Update, 1*(6), 41–43.

Wooten, P. (1996). *Compassionate laughter: Jest for your health!* Salt Lake City, UT: Commune-A-Key Publishing.

CHAPTER 7

Spirituality

THE NATURE OF SPIRITUALITY

Bernie Siegel, physician and author, once threatened to form a group of people who would eat only high-fat meals, learn to smoke, become "couch potatoes," and engage in little or no exercise. Siegel had talked with so many desperately ill people who had experienced a deeply moving, life-changing spirituality during the struggle to cope with the disease, he decided that his little band would seek to develop a terminal illness so they could experience transcendence! Said in humor, he nevertheless hit on a profound truth. No one consciously seeks to be sick, but during illness and dying, sometimes a special kind of inner strength is developed.

There are probably as many definitions of spirituality as there are people. Most definitions incorporate the idea that spirituality includes reaching out from one's inner self both horizontally and vertically. The horizontal dimension refers to a connectedness with others, a "nonreligious sense of life purpose and life satisfaction" (Champagne, 1989). The vertical dimension refers to one's relationship with one's God, the Universe, or of something greater than self. It gives a sense of meaning. Both the horizontal and vertical dimensions transcend, or move beyond, the physical world (see Figure 7-1). A healing relationship involves both dimensions. A healing relationship involves spirituality because it involves connectedness to others and a sense of meaning.

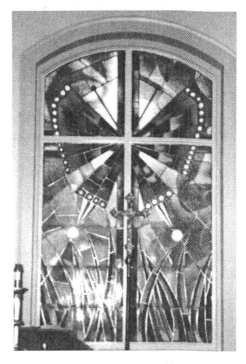

Figure 7-1 Window of a butterfly represents transformation to residents of senior center. *(This window is located at a Rodenberg Chapel, Franke Home, Lutheran Homes of South Carolina, Mount Pleasant, SC.)*

Reducing the concept of spirituality to definitions is an academic exercise that is necessary to study ways of assisting dying people. But somehow definitions of spirituality never seem to capture the real essence of this most beautiful part of human experience. The spirit of a person is what gives meaning to life, integrates body and mind, identifies the individual as unique and as having intrinsic value just for existing. It is part of the mystery of life, requiring us to act morally and responsibly to others as well as to search for the Transcendent. Our spirit energizes and gives us purpose and direction. It makes us whole, unified in all parts of our being. Caring for oneself inescapably involves care of one's spirit.

SPIRITUAL DEVELOPMENT

Westerhoff (1976) believed that spiritual development occurs throughout life, and defined four stages of faith:

- *experienced* faith, occurring in childhood by interaction with others (such as family) of a similar faith tradition
- *affiliative* faith, occurring in late adolescence, developed by actively participating in activities of a faith tradition, such as youth groups, missionary work, meditation groups
- *searching* faith, a part of young adulthood, developed by questioning and searching and doubting one's faith
- *owned* faith, the faith of commitment, a mature faith

Although this is a Eurocentric model, it is useful for its simplicity and parallel structure to psychological development. In this model, the early stages of spiritual growth, or the acquisition of faith, are more focused on the horizontal relationship with family and friends. This parallels social development. As one matures, the vertical component of spirituality develops. Although Westerhoff linked spiritual growth to chronologic stages of development, it is widely acknowledged that spiritual growth may begin and continue to develop at any age.

It is the internal struggle and search for meaning that is so characteristic of young adults that changes the direction of the relationship to a more vertical attribute. One can imagine spiritual development in this stage using the metaphor of a young tree putting roots solidly into the ground. The tree stretches its branches upward, receives warmth from above, and becomes a conduit for the nourishment from the earth to all parts of the tree, and beyond. Like the spiritually mature person, the tree becomes strong, has its own identity, yet is able to support others. The cycle of the seasons, including falling leaves giving way for new buds, suggests continuity of life. Most spiritual traditions include a sense of continuity of life, continuity of the vertical axis of spirituality.

It is possible to develop either the horizontal axis of spirituality or the vertical axis, rather than both. One dying patient became intensely interested in writing a family history. He used his last few months to trace the origins of his family through genealogical charts. He found meaning in his own life in a connectedness to those around him. His place on the family tree was defined through exploring the horizontal aspect of his spirituality. Human relationships were his main interest.

In the early centuries of Christianity, groups of monks sought to develop a relationship with God, and understand the mysteries of life in that way. They were called the Desert Fathers. They spent their lives "striving to re-direct every aspect of body, mind and soul to God" (Ward, 1975). For these men, the vertical relationship between themselves and God was all important. This gave their lives meaning. They were hospitable to travelers and shared their meager supplies with anyone in need, but they did it as service to God, not as connection with people.

SPIRITUAL HEALTH

For most people, spiritual health requires the development of spirituality in both the horizontal and vertical directions throughout the life span. It is not static, but a dynamic ebb and flow of energy that helps one to feel satisfied with life. The National Interfaith Coalition on Aging (NICA) defines spiritual well-being in part as the "affirmation of life in a relationship with God, self, community and environment that nurtures and celebrates wholeness" (Cook, 1980). Seidll (1993) defines spiritual health as "that aspect of our well-being which organizes the values, the relationships, and the meaning and purpose of our lives."

People who have faced a life-threatening illness and learned to live with it peacefully tell of a journey inward, going into a place within themselves where they learn to accept the fact of the illness. This is not resignation or defeat. They find a courage that enables them to embrace life as it is now, a kind of inner wisdom. They decide to live before they die, and set realistic goals for today and tomorrow. One man took part in a race he had always wanted to do, another opened a business. A woman decided to live until her first grandchild was born. In some cases, the illness went into long-term remission. In others, it did not. But each of the people who adopted this attitude talked of dying as "life enhancing" (Kussman, 1993).

When illness and impending death threaten an individual, the self is always threatened. Death threatens the physical continuity of existence. People search for new meaning and understanding for the whole person at that time. Dr. Elizabeth Kübler-Ross suggested that death does not occur in an instant, but is a continuous process throughout life. Therefore, she suggested that people befriend death, see it as a companion along the path of life. She suggested that befriending death allows one to "truly live your life rather than simply pass through it" (Kübler-Ross, 1975). This distinction refers to depth and meaning in life, a spiritual characteristic. If a person has been able to take the advice of Dr. Kübler-Ross, the threat may be less severe. Denial of death, which is common in American society, interferes with a person's ability to befriend death and reach a level of acceptance.

SPIRIT AND MIND

There is a relation between spiritual and psychological health. Because people function as whole, indivisible beings, anyone who has difficulty forming relationships due to a lack of psychological development or psychological problems may not be able to form relationships in the spiritual sense. Part of spirituality is the ability to love and be loved. Caring for the dying person who has a spiritual need and helping that person move toward spiritual health requires caring for that person in the psychological areas of being as well. Excellent communication skills, role-modeling appropriate relationships and connectedness, and establishing trust are mental health skills that are useful in providing spiritual care.

RELIGION AND SPIRITUALITY

Spirituality is a universal human attribute. Everyone is spiritual. Religion is a formal system for the expression of a doctrine or belief. Not everyone has clearly articulated a system of belief, nor joined a religious group. Many people who feel themselves to be spiritual do not admit to being religious. And people who demonstrate an intense religiosity—an outward form of formalized, ritualistic religious behavior, may not appear to be spiritual to others.

Members of many religious groups record a moment of spirituality, perhaps a transcendent moment in a piece of great art, literature, or music, enriching life for all who see or hear it. Stained glass windows,

Tibetan chimes, Christmas cantatas, and chants from a variety of religious traditions are examples. Individuals also record their spiritual depths in great art of all forms. Michelangelo's Pieta and Sufi poetry have the power to move, to reach the inner soul. Those present at a performance or in an artistic milieu resonate together, creating a special bond that helps each one to identify meaning in life from the aesthetic ambience that the authors, artists, or composers created.

Formal religious affiliation serves as an expression of spirituality. It can be a kind of spiritual support group. Shared rituals and rites, and transmission of values through the generations nurture and provide benchmarks of an individual's journey through life. They help establish belongingness and love. The wedding ceremony and funeral services are two examples. Those members of a religious faith who are absent from a planned group meeting or service may feel they are sustained in the memory of the group, and perhaps by prayer. Those who are near death may take comfort in the thought that they will be remembered, both by family and friends, and by their deity.

However, there can be problems within an organized group. Any formally constituted group of people, including church, synagogue, or mosque, has expectations of its members. These expectations may conflict with the way an individual feels. If members of an organized religion believe that death is reunion with God, or a doorway to a new life, and should be viewed as a positive event, the anxiety a dying person feels may be seen as failure to live up to expectations. If that occurs, the patient may choose not to use the group for support, diminishing a useful resource for reducing anxiety and moving toward wholeness.

Clergy can be very helpful in assisting the patient to understand that anxiety and fear are normal, that spirituality does not depend on a certain feeling about one event, and that the religious organization and God are not synonymous. The perceptive nurse or counsellor exercises tact and a special sensitivity with both the clergy and the patient when there is conflict or guilt because of feelings of failure to live up to a perceived standard of behavior. In this case, consultation with the clergy provides open, honest dialogue. A working relationship and mutual respect between health care providers and clergy in the community helps the consultation process.

Some groups have a statement of belief, hold to a commonly accepted statement of values, and invoke a higher power but do not identify themselves as religious organizations. Alcoholics Anonymous and other 12-step self-help programs are examples of such groups because they have expectations and rites based on values and a belief in a higher power, which some equate with religion. Group membership is one form of spirituality, and provides the support needed to grow toward wholeness.

If a person who is dying has expressed spirituality within a religious group, the group may be an important support during the time of dying. Religion as an expression of one's spirituality is a great help to many people, even if they have been away from it for some time.

Mr. Bower and the Priest

It was clear that Mr. Bower had a question. He waited for several hours for Ms. F., who was busy that night. He smoked in the lounge, dozed in a chair in his room, and walked the hall. When the nurse sat down, he called to her and suggested she "take a break" and sit in the day room with him for a few minutes. Recognizing his need to talk, she did so. His question took a few minutes to be asked, but it was simple. "I haven't been to church for 15 years. I used to be Catholic. Would it be fair to call the priest just because I'm dying?" At 3:00 A.M. in a darkened solarium with a lonely man nearing the end of his life, Ms. F. identified the problem as another relationship that needed healing. He discussed his problem of whether to call the priest or not for two weeks. He was not sure it was fair to God, fair to the church, or fair to himself to reopen his connection with formalized religion. After exploring what it meant to him to be fair, he recognized that it was okay to do something for himself based on his own idea of need. Men have needs, too, even veteran military men who have been self-sufficient for most of their lives. The priest was called. Mr. Bower began to work on his relationship with God, and his priest helped him.

SPIRITUAL NEED AND SPIRITUAL DISTRESS

Spiritual need has been defined as "any factors necessary to establish and/or maintain a person's dynamic personal relationship with God (as defined by that individual) and out of that relationship to experience forgiveness, love, hope, trust and meaning and purpose in life" (Stallwood & Stoll, 1975, p. 1088). The North American Nursing Diagnosis Association (1994, p. 49) calls *spiritual distress* "a state in which an individual experiences a disruption in the life principle which pervades a person's entire being and which integrates and transcends one's biological and psychosocial nature." These definitions are useful in the assessment of spiritual needs and the provision of nursing care. They suggest that forgiveness, love, hope, trust, and meaning and purpose in life are necessary to limit disruption in the integrating and transcending force in a person's life. The definitions also suggest that those characteristics are present as a result of a relationship with God (as defined by that individual). The nurse may discover that the key to helping a person in spiritual distress is to find ways to help preserve and restore those qualities, and support an individual's relationship with the divine.

Forgiveness

Mr. Bower wanted to reestablish a connection with his former religious affiliation, but before he could do so, he needed to experience forgiveness. His separation from his church only began to be a problem that he identified toward the end of his life. The reasons for the separation did not really matter. He harbored no anger or memories that made the reunion fearful or awkward. He simply wanted to return. The separation had begun to interfere with his relationship with God. His fear was that others would judge him, or consider him unworthy. Perhaps God would, as well. He felt guilty. A formal reconciliation and reaffirmation of faith was helpful to him.

Spiritual forgiveness is not always a matter of going back to a group. Some people need to be forgiven by their God figure, for a previous wrong (sin); by other people they believe they have wronged; or by themselves. The experience of Joe and Debbi illustrates the point.

Joe and Debbi

Joe and Debbi believed that God had answered their prayers when their young daughter, who had been diagnosed with leukemia, went into remission. When she relapsed and subsequently died, Joe and Debbi lost their faith. They felt betrayed by God who had reneged on a promise. They stopped attending church and denied God's existence. In their anger, they said things to friends about God that they later felt guilty about. Their anger and guilt made reconciliation difficult because they found it hard to forgive themselves for what they had felt and said. Guilt and anger are often signs of the need for forgiveness and spiritual reconciliation.

Forgiveness does not always lead to reconciliation. Neither is forgiveness justifying or condoning harmful actions or violations. It is the voluntary letting go of the right to retaliate after injury. It is an act to let go of pain, resentment, and outrage that you have carried as a burden (Kornfield, 1999). It is taking "seriously the awfulness that has happened when you are treated unfairly" (Tutu, 1999). It is the relinquishing of one's right to anger and resentment in response to an injury (North, 1997). It is a potentially liberating and restoring willful human response to a violation (Festa & Tuck, 2000). For health care teams, forgiveness may be identified as an issue of central significance in patient care and clinical practice, particularly for dying people.

For people who believe they have been harmed or violated by another, the festering of that burden over time leads to anger and bitterness, sometimes self-loathing and harsh internal criticism. This interferes with other relationships, and potentiates a variety of physical problems like hypertension and psychoneuroimmunologic alterations (Festa & Tuck, 2000).

Forgiveness is not easy. Dowrick (1997) lists five qualities a person must have in order to forgive:

- courage: more than bravery

- fidelity: to oneself and one's friends, destiny, beliefs, values, vocation, and one's faith

- restraint: an act of will, an expression of freedom to choose and act

- generosity: the willing giving of your time, interest, concern, care, understanding, humor, loyalty, or honesty

- tolerance: for your own interior chaos and clashes

The nurse's role includes an assessment of the patient's readiness to forgive, to get past their anger. Some may need to feel like a victim or a martyr or have other reasons for not being ready. But when they are ready, the health care team members recognize forgiveness as a process (Enright, 1991; Festa & Tuck, 2000; Worthington, 1998). General questions, like "Is there someone you would like to be closer to?" followed by "What is keeping you from it?" may help the nurse understand the problem. In general, the process should include an awareness of the hurt, a conscious decision to give up the guilt or hurt, and for many, a meeting with the one hurt or doing the hurting, and confession or restitution when possible. The process may take months or years and require interdisciplinary assistance as strong emotion is often evoked.

For the person who is finally able to forgive (or ask forgiveness), the results are peace, and the physical and emotional benefits that accrue as a result of peace. Anger and hostility are reduced, relationships improve, and some physical problems may be lessened. Most importantly, a person is able to get on with the life that is left with less burden.

Hope

Hope is a vital spiritual need. Hope is the willingness to embrace all of life's possibilities. Siegel (1986) suggested that hope is energy, that lack of hope is a wish to die. In this context, the wish to die is not a peaceful letting go of life with tasks completed and planned entry into the mystery of death, but a giving up because it is too hard to live. Hope means that there is a future. Hope is correlated with a feeling of well-being. A general kind of hope for the best life possible under the conditions is as useful as hope that has a more defined goal.

Hope may be specific or nonspecific. Specific things to hope for include:

- some new treatment or drug to prolong life
- physical restoration
- the ability to love and be loved
- reconciliation with something or someone in the past
- finding meaning in the mystery of death
- life after death (Speck, 1993)

Health care providers who tell the patient there is nothing more that can be done interfere with hope. There is always something that can be done in a caring relationship, even if it is only the provision of comfort and relief of pain. Dr. C. Northrup (Kussman, 1993) always tells her patients who have a poor diagnosis/prognosis of the four or five miracles in her patient population, the people who were supposed to die of a disease and did not. It is not ethical to promise cure or anything else that can't be delivered, but it is useful to tell the truth—that some people do live in spite of poor odds. No one knows why. There is hope. This is not to be confused with denial, a refusal to see the possibility of one's death, or to see the signs and do the things necessary to care for one's self given the circumstances present. Hope in this context is to see all the possibilities, including that of life.

There are many things that can interfere with hope. A long parade of strangers who go into and out of a room without really seeing the patient, as in rounds by students from a variety of health care disciplines, may inadvertently give the message that the patient doesn't count any more. People feel that because cure is not foreseen, their case is hopeless but curious. Taking the time to make sure the patient is included in the discussion, and asking about plans and goals for today, give hope. Patients should be partners in the healing process, encouraged to make choices about how to live life now. This is also true for the person at home. If the sick room is entered only when it is time to bring a meal, give a medication or treatment, or other care of some kind, the person becomes isolated, feels like a burden, and becomes hopeless. Family, friends, and other support people need to help the person plan, share thoughts and insights, and hope.

Pity also diminishes hope. It is belittling. The person who pities another doesn't see that person in the fullness of who she is. Only the disease or disability is seen. Patients ought to systematically decrease their contact with people who pity them or otherwise bring them down (Kussman, 1993).

Mr. Kashu (see Chapter 2) gave up hope when he felt betrayed by his son. When family relationships are strained and not working, loss of hope can be the result. All the things done to support family relationships while a person is close to death assist to maintain hope.

Trust

People who feel abandoned at a critical time get angry. If the illness that is likely to end in death is the reason for the anger, the angry behavior may be aimed at the nurse. The same techniques for handling anger in other settings are useful, including helping the patient to identify the anger and the reason for the anger; setting appropriate limits on destructive behavior; and, most importantly, using honesty, presence, and genuine caring to help develop a sense of trust. Trust is like the support for the bridge of reconciliation that allows an individual to move from a land of isolation, anger, guilt, and fear to a land where relationships, love, hope, and meaning can exist.

The ability to trust is learned early in life, and if it is not, an individual probably has had difficulty with relationships throughout life. A history of having had at least a few long-lasting relationships in life is helpful information in assessing a patient's ability to trust in the present time. A person who feels abandoned and who is no longer able to trust others feels powerless, empty, afraid, and possibly out of control. The nurse who gives the patient reason to trust by providing clear and accurate information, appropriate reassurance, and some control over the treatment process is giving spiritual care.

Meaning

Frankl (1952) suggested other characteristics of spirituality that can be lived within a group or individually. Three areas of values that give meaning to people who are suffering are the opportunity to create or achieve tasks; the ability to experience goodness, truth, beauty, or a significant relationship; and the choice of attitude a person takes toward the suffering. Frankl studied spirituality in relation to survival of the concentration camp experience during World War II. Survivors of the camps were the people who could find a weed along the road and see beauty in it, remember a spouse with great tenderness, and even laugh at how they were beginning to smell when the soap ran out. The attitude that led to making a joke of tragedy seems to be lifesaving. It certainly helps one to experience life more fully.

Neither spirituality nor its expression through religion means that people will remain healthy or avoid suffering. Saints and sinners alike suffer and die. Dossey (1993, p. 34) warned against healers who recommend specific techniques to "transform one's personality, relationships, goals, thought habits, philosophy, and overall orientation to life" in order to achieve certain specific results. No one has shown that terminal illness is a result of imperfection in the way a person thinks, or that if a person can straighten out grievances against others and learn to love or relate to others in a different way, the disease will miraculously disappear. Changing one's relationships and becoming more open should be things a person chooses to do for the sake of the relationship, to meet the felt need of connecting with others so that life is more satisfying now, not for the purpose of avoiding or curing suffering or illness.

Spirituality is not something sought, but something that is. Behaviors and attitudes are manifestations of the spiritual life. Vietnamese Buddhist Priest Thich Nhat Hanh writes of suffering during the worst days of the war. "In that intense suffering, you feel a kind of relief and joy within yourself, because you know that you are an instrument of compassion. Understanding such intense suffering and realizing compassion in the midst of it, you become a joyful person, even if your life is very hard." (Hanh, 1991, p. 125). One can imagine that this gentle monk lived in all three of the areas that Frankl said gave meaning in suffering. He had tasks to do as a result of his compassion; saw goodness, truth, and relationship where he was; and cultivated an attitude of peace in the face of suffering.

SPIRITUAL ASSESSMENT

It is not easy to assess a person's spiritual health or spiritual distress. The interrelationship of psychological and spiritual behaviors like anger mean that assessment of one gives insight into the other. Stoll (1979) listed four specific areas of assessment of spiritual concerns:

- one's concept of God or deity
- source of strength and hope
- significance of religious practices and rituals
- perceived relationship of spiritual beliefs and state of health

During an interview, each of these areas can be assessed using direct questions. Simple questions asking if a God figure or religion is important in a person's life, what one's concept of the deity is, or if prayer is useful help develop insights about that person's spiritual focus. Knowing what things or people gave spiritual strength in the past, what religious practices and rituals give comfort now, and how each of those things affects the person's perceived state of health can form the basis of a plan to assure continued spiritual care based on a person's own choices.

Even without a formal interview, patients can suggest that they are experiencing some degree of spiritual distress. If they talk about a diety or other spiritual topics, even in a lighthearted fashion, this may reveal the fact that much thought is going on regarding their relationship to their own spirituality or faith. Comments about religious functions a patient cannot attend, negative results of prayer, or rejection of clergy all may indicate spiritual distress.

Nonverbal behaviors also may indicate spiritual distress. Some of those behaviors reflect concurrent psychological and physical distress because a sad spirit results in a distressed person. These are some behaviors that may indicate spiritual distress:

- expressions of anger (toward God or others)
- sleep disturbances
- increased discomfort in the absence of obvious cause
- inconsistent mood (crying, withdrawal, anxiety)
- restlessness
- social isolation
- gallows humor
- preoccupation with questions about meaning of life, God, or suffering
- rejection of people from one's spiritual heritage or background (Carson, 1989)

Assessment of the environment also aids in the plan for spiritual care. There may be religious books, medals, icons, get-well cards with a religious motif, or music that family or friends have brought to comfort a person. A very restless, semicomatose dying man visibly relaxed when a family member played a tape of the music performed at the service the last Saturday the man had been present at his synagogue. That kind of observation is helpful in planning care. However, the nurse must be careful not to overinterpret symbols or behaviors without asking the patient. A book on prayer may be present as a well-meant gift from a friend that the patient has no intention of reading, and no interest in. The fact that the patient has a friend who sends such a book may be more important.

NURSING INTERVENTIONS

Nowhere is the need for healing relationships more important than for the person in spiritual distress. The goal of care for the person in spiritual distress is to assist that person to experience forgiveness, love, trust, hope, and a sense of meaning and purpose in life, based on a dynamic relationship with God (as that person identifies the relationship).

The Nurse

For a nurse who undertakes to help a person in spiritual distress, Carson (1989, p. 21) has some good advice.

> Each nurse needs to acknowledge his or her own personal spiritual journey, for it is in the continuous meeting of one's own spiritual needs that one will know the meaning of spiritual well-being. The greatest gift the nurse has to give to clients is one's personal, living, spiritual richness. This gift of one's true self given in care to the client experiencing crisis will inevitably encourage the client toward spiritual well-being.

The nurse's own spirituality will be reflected in the choice of interventions selected. The interventions selected will be based in part on skills discussed in previous chapters, like the communication skills of active listening, reflection, and clarification, or presence, the sense of being fully focused in this moment for this individual. In addition, the nurse who feels secure in spiritual matters may demonstrate a sense of empathy, humility, and commitment.

Empathy requires that one is able to feel in some degree what the patient is feeling, and to be able to put it into words, so that it can be examined by the person. No one feels exactly as another person does, so it is inaccurate to say, "I know how you feel." But a nurse may be able to say, "I'd probably be angry, too, if I were dying before I felt like I was ready. Let's discuss some things we might do that would help you feel better, to get ready." From this discussion, it might be possible to determine resources and strengths the patient might use and relationships to call on that would alleviate some of the distress.

Humility allows both the client and the nurse to accept each other as finite human beings who don't know all the answers (Carson, 1989, p. 168). The nurse is fully competent in nursing care and able to provide comfort, pain control, and appropriate treatments, but the choices of direction in the client's life, including the meaning of that life, are determined by the client. The nurse simply provides opportunity, environment, and support as needed so that the spiritual journey can be experienced. Commitment is the choice to share the journey with the client for a little while. It means to make one's self available when a patient needs support, even when it is hard to do so. It is often hard to maintain a relationship with a patient through a terminal illness and be present when that person dies. To be committed to sharing this experience with a patient requires that the nurse maintain a healthy spirituality and support system. Chapter 11 gives suggestions for helping nurses and other caregivers maintain their own health in situations that require a great deal of love and giving of self.

Spiritual Help for the Dying

There are at least five very specific things that can be helpful for the spiritual care of the person who is dying. They include: prayer, presence of loved ones, a time to share, assisting the person to finish any business or things still to be accomplished, and giving permission to die.

Prayer and meditation may be a part of religious experience that some people would like to share. For the person who meditates regularly, provision for a period of time without interruption and perhaps for some physical support to help the person maintain his regular meditative position (like sitting in a particular posture) are indicated. For those who pray, a loved one, clergy, or the nurse may choose to share prayer, if it would be comforting. Provision for quiet and privacy should be made. It may be helpful to agree beforehand on the kind of prayer or meditation, so both people involved are comfortable with the arrangements. Prayer can take many forms, so it is important to ask the person about what is comfortable. A familiar prayer that holds special significance or is offered at a particular time may be comforting. For example, a child may be comforted and feel connected with home and family as well as God if assisted to continue a traditional family prayer such as "Now I lay me down to sleep, I pray the Lord my soul to keep; if I should die before I wake, I pray the Lord my soul to take." Prayer and meditation assist a person to maintain trust in something beyond self, a spiritual relationship.

Dossey called prayer "nonlocal healing" in some instances, and pointed out that many studies have shown that even when a person does not know she is being prayed for, the person being prayed for may feel better. Nonspecific prayers, such as "Thy will be done," may be more effective than goal-oriented prayer for a specified outcome (Dossey, 1993). He and others make a clear and well-documented case for the fact that prayer helps (Meisenhelder & Chandler, 2000). Carson (1989, p. 169) says that through prayer "the individual communicates needs, feelings, fears, love, adoration, and awe to the Creator. In return, God graces the person with a sense of his presence and his abiding love."

The presence of people significant in one's life is important for spiritual well-being. The nature of one's healing relationship with one's own diety or spirituality, including the sense of forgiveness, love, and meaning, is reflected in one's relationship with significant people in life. Limiting visiting hours, especially at the time close to death, is not helpful unless there is a clear reason for it for the patient's well-being. There are many stories, some well-documented, of a loved one appearing at the bedside of a patient in the moments just before death. The loved one seemed to know that death was near, even without having been called to the bedside. The connection between the two people was maintained even at a distance.

Grandpa John

Grandpa John was dying, and the end was near. His breathing was labored, and he appeared to be waiting. His family had been called to come to the hospital. The student nurse was sitting at the bedside. Looking out of the window, he saw the old man's family drive up in their battered, well-used car. He told Grandpa John that the family was here. The man looked at the student, smiled, closed his eyes, took one last breath, and died. The student told the family their grandpa had waited for them, and he knew the family had come. That news was comforting to the family. The old man had waited until he had done all he could for his loved ones. Grandpa John had waited to die until his family had come to the hospital, and the fact of their presence gave him permission to die.

People need private time to share. If they participate in rites, such as sacraments or special observances, the time and place should be respected. A visit to the outside of the building may be necessary to see the sun or feel the breeze. This sometimes is a spiritual experience for the person who finds spirituality in a connection with nature. The person with whom the patient shares this experience, a sibling, parent, spouse, or friend, should be encouraged and assisted. The nurse advocates for the patient's right to maintain spiritual connectedness in any way that is useful to the patient and does not interfere with the rights of others.

Many people seem to wait for permission to die. A child dying of a long-term genetic disease had talked of going to be with God. But on the day that he was so close to death that he was struggling for every breath, he did not die until his mother told him, "I think it is time for you to be with God." His struggles ceased, he was comforted, and he died later that day. His mother had given him peace by giving him permission to die.

SUMMARY

During the course of dying, some people turn toward an inner wisdom that helps them transform the experience from fear, anger, loss, or sense of catastrophe to an ability to embrace all of life. The relationships with family and loved ones deepen and are characterized by forgiveness, trust, love, and an abiding sense of satisfaction and purpose that has been fulfilled. They feel the presence of their God, the universal, the meaning beyond self. Sometimes the nurse is privileged to support the patient through these changes. Providing an environment and resources to allow a person to pursue spiritual development is a part of spiritual care. Assessing for spiritual distress and becoming an avenue of communication in order to support relationships are critical in the relief of spiritual distress and in helping the dying person choose to live fully in the remaining time.

However, the nurse who shares the experience with the patient, who gives of self in presence, humility, empathy, and commitment, shares the satisfaction of a mature spirituality. The nurse cares for self while caring for the patient, and grows in grace and the comfort of healing relationships.

REFERENCES

Carson, V. (1989). *Spiritual dimensions of nursing practice.* Philadelphia: W.B. Saunders.

Champagne, K. (1989). Value-belief pattern. In G. McFarland & E. McFarland (Eds.), *Nursing diagnosis & prevention: Planning for patient care.* St. Louis, MO: C.V. Mosby Co.

Cook, T. C. (1980). Preface. In J. A. Thorson & T. C. Cook (Eds.), *Spiritual well-being of the elderly.* Springfield, IL: Charles C. Thomas.

Dossey, L. (1993). *Healing words.* San Francisco: HarperCollins.

Dowrick, S. (1997). *Forgiveness and other acts of love.* Victoria, Australia: Penguin Books.

Enright, R. D. (1991). The human development study group. The moral development of forgiveness. In W. Kurines, & J. Gewirtz (Eds.), *Moral behavior and development,* Vol. 1. Hillsdale, NJ: Erlbaum, 123–152.

Festa, L. M., & Tuck, I. (2000). A review of forgiveness literature with implications for nursing practice. *Holistic Nursing Practice, 14*(4), 77–86.

Frankl, V. (1952). *The doctor and the soul.* New York: Bantam Books.

Hanh, T. (1991). *Peace is every step.* New York: Bantam Books.

Kornfield, J. (1999). An act of the heart. *Spirituality and Health,* Winter, 29.

Kübler-Ross, E. (1975). *Death: The final stage of growth.* Englewood Cliffs, NJ: Prentice Hall.

Kussman, L. (Producer) (1993). *Harbor of hope.* [Videotape] (Available from Aquarius Productions, Inc., 35 Main St., Wayland, MA 01778).

Meisenhelder, J. B., & Chandler, E. N. (2000). Prayer and health outcomes in church members. *Alternative Therapies in Health and Medicine, 6*(4), 56–60.

North American Nursing Diagnosis Association. (1994). *Taxonomy I* (rev. 1990). St. Louis, MO: NANDA.

North, J. (1997). Wrongdoing and forgiveness. *Philosophy, 61,* 499–508.

Seidll, L. G. (1993). The value of spiritual health. *Health Progress,* September, 49.

Siegel, B. (1986). *Love, medicine, and miracles.* New York: Harper & Row.

Speck, P. (1993). Spiritual issues in palliative care. In D. Doyle, G. W. C. Hanks, & N. MacDonald (Eds.), *Oxford textbook of palliative medicine.* Oxford: Oxford University Press.

Stallwood, J., & Stoll, R. (1975). Spiritual dimensions of nursing practice. In I. L. Beland & H. Y. Passos (Eds.), *Clinical Nursing* (3rd ed.). New York: McMillan.

Stoll, R. (1979). Guidelines for spiritual assessment. *American Journal of Nursing, 9,* 1574.

Tutu, D. (1999). *Spirituality and Health,* Winter, 29.

Ward, B. (1975). *The sayings of the desert fathers.* Kalamazoo, MI: Cistercian Publications.

Westerhoff, J. (1976). *Will our children have faith?* New York: Seabury Press.

Worthington, E. (1998). An empathy-humility-commitment model of forgiveness applied with family dyads. *Journal of Family Therapy, 20,* 59–76.

PART
III

Help for Families

CHAPTER
8

Families

GOALS

Families provide the primary social support for many sick people. Resources in terms of care, transportation, activities of daily living, and social interaction generally start with the family. But not all families are prepared to provide this support.

Mrs. Peterson's family met her physical needs for nutrition, hygiene, pain control, and safety. But she was not emotionally connected to the people around her who had given her life meaning. Mrs. Peterson had been the kind of Mom who baked cookies, went to the PTA, and served as room mother for each of her three children's fourth-grade classes. She had entertained her husband's clients and was on the board of the local recreation department. In this final illness, it seemed she was still serving others by not bothering them, which was her long-time pattern of behavior.

Mrs. Gage knew that this was a family in trouble. Unless healing occurred, unless family members and Mrs. Peterson could begin to talk about the future, the family would probably have difficulty grieving later, perhaps experiencing guilt, tension, and prolonged grief. Mrs. Peterson would not be assured of her impact on the lives of others, or of her place in their memories. She might not have the opportunity to say good-bye, to release them from a continued sense of obligation ("I should have done more"), or to do some of the practical tasks for the family that make life easier after the death of a loved one. This family needed help to

Mrs. Peterson

Mrs. Peterson clearly had difficulty moving around, but she told the hospice nurse that she tried not to call her family for help unless she really had to. She had her own bedroom in the eight-room home that was neat and well-kept. There was a television with remote control and a variety of care aids, including the hospital bed in which she slept. Several times during the assessment visit, Mrs. Gage, the hospice nurse, noted family members in the hall passing the bedroom door. They never said anything or even appeared to look into the room. One young son, a teenager, brought lemonade about 30 minutes into the visit, but did not stay. Mrs. Peterson excused the behavior, saying they were busy and did not have much time to stop and talk. When the nurse asked her why they had waited until so late in the course of her illness to contact hospice, Mrs. Peterson said that they had been managing, and the eldest son who did not live in the home was opposed to hospice. It had taken him until now to permit the call.

Mrs. Gage assessed the situation. Mrs. Peterson was effectively isolated, socially unavailable. Her family provided for physical needs, medications, and entertainment opportunities. They would provide a videotape for entertainment, but would not stay with her to watch it. They seemed uncomfortable around her. When they were not in the home, her friends could not get into the house, so they stopped dropping by. She did some visiting by telephone. The family members meant well, but they led busy lives, and did not recognize that they had a limited time with the wife and mother. They were not dealing with their own feelings about the situation. Talking with the elder son, a professional man who happened to come into the house at the end of the visit, Mrs. Gage asked him why he had been opposed to hospice care. He frankly answered that calling hospice meant that they had given up, that his mother would die. It seemed that by avoiding the call they would avoid the death.

share the truth of the impending death and what it would mean to them all. If they could share the truth, tension in the home would decrease and a sense of completion of the relationship might be achieved.

Goals of the health care team in this circumstance include:

1. Maintain and support the physical care being given.

2. Increase the numbers of visits to the room for social reasons by helping the family find ways to visit or let friends into the house on a regular schedule.

3. Help the family to begin to talk about Mrs. Peterson's death and its meaning for them.

4. Help Mrs. Peterson to remain connected to her family in spite of their reluctance to discuss serious issues.

5. Make sure Mrs. Peterson has the opportunity to plan for her own future through advance directives, wills, and other legal needs.

CONNECTING

Emotional cutoff (remaining emotionally distant or being unwilling to maintain a relationship at an emotional level) may be both the reason and the result of the inability of the family to talk with each other about an impending death. Generally, as tension in the home (or place where the dying person and family meet) increases, anxiety increases. This leads to deteriorating relationships, explosive outbursts or withdrawal, poor choices and lack of planning for care (especially of self), and eventually a hopelessness or depression. Chapter 6 gives some useful techniques for helping people to deal with anxiety.

Long-term illness complicates relationships. If people do not discuss feelings, it seems that everyone involved is living a lie, enacting a sham existence. A patient who may wish for such things as reconciliation with an estranged child, a divorced mate, or an old classmate cannot have them because "the family would not understand" and the topic is taboo. Everyone is protecting everyone else from the truth because the truth hurts, but the results of not living in the truth are separation, isolation, emotional pain, and lack of resolution of the problems. Protecting another from bad news is paternalism.

When a nurse meets a patient who has a suspected terminal diagnosis, it is important to recognize two components of the healing role. The nurse is a role model in truth telling and a patient advocate with the family, the health care team, the institution, and society. This role does not pit the nurse and patient against everyone else. It is likely that everyone involved wants the best for the patient. Creating opportunities for open communication (but not forcing it) will help the group and the patient achieve the best, whatever that is determined to be.

Truth Telling

The Peterson family needed to begin telling each other (and themselves) the truth about why they walk by Mrs. Peterson's room without calling out a hello or dropping in to visit now and then. Mrs. Peterson needed to be able to tell them that she would like them to visit more often, and perhaps share some entertainment or just talk. After beginning to share a few moments, they needed to acknowledge the fact that Mrs. Peterson was dying and some plans had to be made.

Mrs. Gage made a start in helping the family to talk when she asked the son why they called hospice so late. He was able to give an honest and perceptive answer. Many families are not able to admit that death within a defined period of time is probable. This son is moving beyond that stage. Other than denial, reasons why families may not be able to share the truth of an impending death with each other include:

- They have a long history of being unable to share with each other about most things.
- They fear the truth will upset the patient.
- They have insufficient information and do not understand that death is even a possibility.
- Their own feelings about death cause them great anxiety.

A family that has a long history of not sharing with each other, that simply has never communicated, is a challenge for the nurse. It is never easy to break a pattern, but during this most important time in people's lives, there may be an opening that can create new patterns of relationships that are more whole and healthy than previous patterns. This can become a kind of legacy from the one who dies to those who remain in a deeper relationship. Mr. Bower was one who had that experience. Professional counseling is often required to achieve this, and referrals aimed at improving a dysfunctional family's communication patterns should be available to the dying patient and family, just as it is to others.

Mr. Bower Had a Daughter

There was no record of a family for Mr. Bower. He considered his veteran friends his family. It was assumed that he spent his weekend passes with a distant relative, perhaps a cousin or uncle. So, when he told Ms. F. about his estranged daughter, she was surprised. By the time he brought it up, he was quite ill. He was ambulatory, but needed regular pain medication in increasing doses, and he tired easily during routine activities like the morning bath ritual.

He had not talked with his daughter for 20 years, but he had gotten her address and wanted to make contact. He was afraid to do so, afraid of rejection. In his postwar years, he had become a heavy drinker and had abandoned his wife and young daughter. He didn't believe that deathbed reunions had fairy tale endings with everyone experiencing a bittersweet reconciliation, and living happily ever after. But in his search for meaning, he had come to believe that he had done one significant thing in his life, and that was to serve his country during the war. Now he wanted to share that one good thing with his daughter by leaving his medals to her after he died. He wanted Ms. F. to tell him how to do it. Should he call his daughter and tell her what was happening, and risk her refusal to accept his precious gift, the meaning of his life? Should he just have them sent after he died, hoping that she would appreciate them? Was there a course of action between these two roads? Should he just leave his medals to his American Legion Post, and forget the long latent hope of reconciliation?

Ms. F. knew that Mr. Bower had developed good coping skills, and that although rejection by the daughter would be painful, he could cope if he had support. She encouraged him to talk with the staff psychologist to plan the phone call, and promised to be available after he called his daughter. As he had expected, there was to be no joyous reunion. The daughter chose not to visit, but she did appreciate the effort he had made to locate her, and was gracious about the medals, promising to pass them on to the grandson Mr. Bower had never met. Mr. Bower was happy he had called, and the two talked twice more before he died. He knew he would be remembered in the next generation. It was enough.

In some cultures, particularly in the Orient, not telling the patient the diagnosis and poor prognosis is expected behavior. The health care community and the society from which it comes believe that it is useful to protect the patient from potentially devastating news because it may lead to hopelessness and loss of the will to live. But in the United States, Kübler-Ross (1969) wrote of many cases that indicate that the dying patient can handle the "awesome truth" when it is delivered with sensitivity, warmth, and directness. The awesome truth includes how loved ones will be affected, how one is likely to die, and all the other questions to which a person needs an answer. Protecting a person has more to do with rapport, communication skills, the ability to demonstrate caring, and timing than it does with the message (Livingston & Williamson, 1985). Only when the truth is shared does the family realize that the time available for saying "I love you" is limited.

Telling the truth includes giving as much information as the patient and family want, when they want it. Postponing information should only be done when it is clear in the professional judgment of the nurse based on sound patient assessment that the information will be damaging. For example, the nurse will call a team meeting or consult with a physician if an AIDS patient confides that when T-lymphocyte counts reach 200, he plans to commit suicide, and the new results now reflect those levels. The patient will still be told what the results are, but with caution and by the person best able to handle the consequences of the information. Truth in this case would include the fact that the patient had mentioned suicide before, and the nurse wants to know if it is still being considered. The patient may be surprised to still feel reasonably well at this stage, and find there is no reason to end life now. There are still goals to be accomplished. Conversely, the patient may still be considering suicide, and in asking about it, the nurse can initiate helpful interventions, like getting a commitment from the patient not to do anything about suicide until he can talk with the psychiatric liaison nurse or the staff psychiatrist or psychologist.

When truth and honesty are shared, the dying patient may have a change in attitude about the meaning of life and what to do with the time left. It is no longer necessary to spend time and energy hiding thoughts from loved ones and avoiding certain topics in conversation. Loved ones can also make plans, access resources like support groups, memorial services, Make-a-wish Foundation, and so on, and say what they want to say now.

Sometimes it happens that the family never feels comfortable enough to share feelings with the dying person before the death. But the sick individual wants to say good-bye and to leave other messages. These kinds of wishes can be fulfilled with creative use of communications skills and a little planning. A lawyer can help with family financial planning and write a will that includes special bequests to special people. A tape recorder or video camera can be used to record thoughts and messages to be heard after the death, or kept for years until small children reach a certain age and messages are meaningful. A diary of a grandmother included several years of day-by-day routine. It was a great comfort to the family later to realize how many friends had called, how often people shoveled the snow from her sidewalk or ran errands while the family felt guilty for not being there more often. After reading the diary, they knew she led a rich and full life, loved them and the things they accomplished, and had realized that those accomplishments could only occur in the distant city in which the children and grandchildren lived. Through the diary, she absolved them of guilt, a great gift.

The terminally ill patient and family need the truth from each other and from health care professionals. The truth shared compassionately and realistically does several things. It

- decreases anxiety for patient and family.
- demonstrates respect and promotes rapport.
- provides information for everyone involved.
- allows the patient to make decisions for self-care.
- provides time for planning.
- gives time for the family to gather support.
- gives time to achieve resolution of end of life issues.

The same results of truth telling are experienced by groups of people who relate to each other around a social issue they work on together, or an intellectual interest, or other common bond. A well-known and much beloved nurse theorist, Dr. Martha Rogers, understood the importance of dealing with death honestly and openly. She had a date to speak to a conference that bore her name—the Rogerian Society. But she also knew she was dying and was not sure she would get to the conference. She did die before the conference, but she had made a tape to play for those gathered there. She used it to say good-bye to many people who had followed her work and admired her greatly. When it was played, it was a moving moment, allowing those present to celebrate the woman and support each other in their loss.

Advocacy

Although there are many definitions of patient advocacy, they all include two components. Advocacy involves giving relevant information and supporting the decisions made by the patient. Advocacy is based on the moral right of people to self-determination. Two of the three characteristics Gadow (1980) used to describe advocacy based on the principle of the right to self-determination are:

1. the nurse's assistance to individuals in exercising their right to self-determination, through decisions that express the full and unique complexity of their values, and

2. a mode of involvement with patients that necessarily engages the entire self of the nurse. (p. 97)

The complexity of values includes those of the whole family and they must be involved in decision making. When any family member is dying, the whole family is changed. Yet, all of the values must be respected, discussed, and shared before satisfying decisions that are right for the whole group are achieved.

This kind of involvement with the family requires the same kinds of characteristics of the nurse as were discussed previously: knowledge of family theory, communication skills, presence, genuineness, and caring. These characteristics help the nurse to assess, plan, and implement the kinds of care that help the family members to make their own decisions, to act on those decisions, and to remain committed to each other.

Commitment to decisions is necessary if the family is to support them. Sometimes, choices that the patient makes can cause the family sorrow, anger, and guilt unless they understand why the decision was made and share in it. For example, if the patient has left final plans that include cremation of the body, and some family members have religious beliefs that prohibit this, conflict will result. Understanding that this is the patient's last wish, and carrying it out as an act of love in spite of one's personal objections can be healing for the family.

The nurse does not get into the position of rescuing the patient, making decisions for the patient or family when they are capable of making them (Donahue, 1985). In Mrs. Peterson's case, the nurse does not become the messenger between Mrs. Peterson and her family. She may suggest that family visit more often, but Mrs. Peterson will decide if she really wants that, and it would be appropriate for Mrs. Peterson to ask the family to do so. If the nurse does that, she may find that she gets one message from the family and a different one from Mrs. Peterson. She may become caught in the middle of a struggle of two groups trying desperately to meet goals of which the other is unaware. It may be helpful to take on the role of facilitator, helping the family and patient to talk with each other. She may role play with Mrs. Peterson, giving her some words to use or ways to ask the family to come in more often. The nurse may be available to the family to answer questions and help them deal with their feelings, but ultimately she must respect their right not to do so if that is what they decide.

Mrs. Peterson needs to be free to make decisions about her own care and relationships without pressure, even if they are in conflict with those of her family. At some point, it is her decision whether to go to a hospital or stay at home with a willing caregiver; about when to stop treatment; and about what she needs to do to maintain the best kind of life for herself for as long as she can. She actively defines the relationship she has with her family. The nurse actively supports these decisions.

Active support for decisions occasionally requires skills in confrontation and negotiation with people or groups outside the family. When hospital or organizational policy prohibits patient choice, the policy is examined for need and relevancy. If it does not serve the safety and patient care needs of others, it may be reviewed to see if it can safely be abrogated. Rigid visiting policies are examples of rules that should be suspended in the interests of patients' rights.

More often than policy problems, intervention is needed because values conflict. The health care system continues to try to preserve life even when the patient may be willing to let go. The nurse who serves as patient advocate must have personal values clearly in mind, and support the patient's right of self-determination. That is not the same thing as agreeing with the decision. Advocacy does not mean that one agrees with the decision made, only with the patient's right to make it. That extends to all of the decisions the patient makes, so long as they do not violate the rights of others or the laws of society. Some nurses are willing to work in the policy or political arenas to bring about social change as a method of patient advocacy.

Caregivers in the role of patient advocate also must intervene if the quality of care rendered is lacking. A patient may have a legitimate complaint about care if it includes: rude behavior from a staff member; failure of staff to respond to a potential threat to life, such as respiratory distress; unresponsiveness of medical team to honor wishes; or, having to wait more than five minutes for pain medication when pain is severe (McFarlane & Bashe, 1998). Advocates with hospitalized patients should know how to make a complaint. First, deal with the person who caused the problem. If that does not get results, go to the supervisor, then the primary physician or hospital ombudsman. Be tactful, have the facts straight, but be firm. One hospital chaplain, visiting a patient recently transferred to a nursing home, assessed substandard care and went to the state agency that licensed the home to complain. He got action!

LEGAL ASPECTS

Advocacy for the patient includes supporting the individual and family in self-determination of treatment choices. There are many reasons why people may not choose the kind of care they want at the end of life. Sometimes they cannot decide because they do not have all the information. They may not have discussed the choices fully with family, and believe that the preferred choice will hurt family members in some way. Some people do not realize that there are choices to be made. They may be in denial. They may go along with each treatment option as it is presented, believing that the health care team knows the right thing to do at each step in the course of the care. Toward the end of a long period of illness, a patient may become very tired and turn inward. He may find discussion or visits with even the most beloved of family to be an intrusion. In those cases, if treatment options have not been discussed previously, they may be left to a trusted colleague or relative. Internal factors limiting the exercise of the right to self-determination of treatment options include:

- inadequate information
- belief that preferred treatment options will hurt family members because of conflicting beliefs
- denial or other emotional factors
- faith that the health care team knows best
- fatigue
- focus on inner issues rather than care

There are also factors external to the dying person that conspire against self-determination of treatment options. When a person is in an environment or among caregivers who believe that the goal is to avoid death at all costs, it is difficult to call a halt to more tests, more drugs, more assessments. If the physician, the nurse, or family members believe that everything possible should be done to prolong life, it is hard for the patient, who is sick, tired, and in pain, to say, "No—I have had enough. I want to focus on comfort, saying good-bye, and peace. It's my time, and I am ready."

Organizations have policies that also affect one's right to make decisions about the end of life. Often based in financial considerations and the laws and regulations of the state and federal government, institutions try to protect themselves from litigation or losing large amounts of money in the care of the dying patient. In one state, a hospital refused to allow the removal of a feeding tube for a patient who was dying even though she had requested that it be removed. The hospital based the decision on potential harm to the patient. They may have feared litigation by family members after the death, or being cited by accrediting bodies for unsafe practice. In this case, transfer of the patient to another state with less restrictive laws allowed the patient to choose the preferred care. In other cases, transfer may be unrealistic because of the patient's condition or costs involved. Referral to the hospital ethics committee allows a full hearing of the issues involved. A full hearing may lead to a legally defensible resolution of the issue in the patient's best interest.

Another case involved the refusal of the patient's family to be responsible for the continued costs of mechanical ventilation as the precipitating factor in getting the hospital administration to allow the ventilator to be turned off according to the patient's wishes. On occasion, a patient who is receiving treatment and is insured privately represents a financial gain to the institution, as when a privately insured patient who is stable but dying a prolonged death is on life-support systems. Factors external to the dying person and family that interfere with the patient's ability to decide the course of treatment include:

- environment in which the goals are always to avoid death at any cost

- personal beliefs of health care professionals or family members that are different from the patient's beliefs
- institutional policies
- state laws and regulations
- reimbursement rates and methods of payment

Advanced Directives

The Patient Self-Determination Act, which went into effect in 1991, requires that all persons who receive funds from Medicare or Medicaid for the care of patients must inform those patients on admission to their services about the right to accept or refuse treatment, and the right to make advanced directives. Advanced directives are legal documents that list those things the patient does not want done in the event he can no longer make decisions for himself (a living will), or gives the right to make decisions about health care to one or more individuals under the same conditions (durable power of attorney for health care). Most organizations offering health care services to the dying now offer standard forms for advanced directives if the patient does not have one already made at the time of admission. These are offered to all people, not only those with Medicare reimbursement (Dunn, 1994).

Standard forms for living wills do not always list everything a patient might wish to include. It is acceptable and in some situations to be encouraged that a person handwrite on the form the additional things requested. It is important to recognize that the person has the right to use this format to request treatment, not just to limit it. For example, a patient may request that care specifically include hydration and nutrition by any means, pain relief, and treatment aimed at maximal comfort. Another example is a patient who may wish to be resuscitated up to three times (if possible) before abandoning those kinds of efforts. Patients do not have the right to demand treatment from those unable or unwilling to provide care they believe is medically futile. For example, if a cardiac arrest occurs and is unwitnessed, and the patient is found dead sometime later, starting CPR would be foolish even if the patient had wished it.

Many people do not have advanced directives. One reason may be that the standard forms have a readability level above the average reading level of patients (Ott & Hardie, 1997). When forms for advanced directives are used, the nurse or other person assisting the patient to fill out the form must be quite clear in the directions, and take care to be sure the form is understood.

Another reason why people do not have advanced directives is that they do not know when or how to get forms and don't believe that they will be followed even if they do fill them out. A nonprofit group, Aging with Dignity, created a document meant to be filled out around the kitchen table with loved ones. It is called "Five Wishes." The people filling it out work through major issues point by point (Chatzky, 2000). Those points include:

- Who will make health care decisions when you cannot?
- What medical treatments are or are not wanted?
- Do you want pain medicine even if it makes you drowsy?
- How and where do you want to be treated? At home? In a hospital?
- What do you want your family and friends to know about you?

Currently, documents using this approach are valid in 34 states. The organization can be reached at 1-888-5wishes.

The living will may be used to limit treatment. A list of treatments often limited by those who are dying includes:

- mechanical ventilation
- cardiopulmonary resuscitation
- invasive diagnostic tests
- antibiotics for infections
- surgical procedures (include or exclude those used for pain control, such as sympathectomy)
- tube feeding
- dialysis
- intravenous infusion
- blood

Some people prefer not to list options about the specific treatments to be allowed or disallowed if they are unable to make decisions for themselves. They prefer to make decisions on a day-to-day basis for as long as possible, and then ask someone they trust to continue making the decisions as they see fit. A durable power of attorney for health care is a legal document giving the right to make those decisions to a named person or a prioritized list of people (e.g., spouse, eldest child, youngest child, aunt, in that order). Asking a person to make those kinds of life-and-death decisions is a huge act of trust, and confers a great responsibility on the person named. The person taking the responsibility should be fully informed of the patient's beliefs about treatment at the end of life and feel comfortable that she knows what the patient would want. The need for clear communication between the two, and belief systems that allow the patient's choices to be fulfilled without violating the decision maker's conscience, is obvious.

A living will may be changed at any time. A nurse who is present when a patient expresses a wish to change the components of a living will has an obligation to report that and to provide the means to do so in writing. Oral statements are legally binding in most states, but should be heard by more than one person. The organization generally has someone familiar with advanced directives who can provide new forms or help a patient alter the old ones. Hospital chaplains and social workers often perform this role. Some states require the changes be notarized.

Prudent people make advanced directives long before the need arrives, even before any diagnosis of illness. People who are dying often believe they know how much time they have and procrastinate about writing the advanced directive. Even those with terminal diagnoses have no guarantee about life tomorrow. A person living at home with a terminal disease can be treated in a trauma center for injuries received in an automobile accident sustained on the way to the doctor's office. The trauma team will not know that the advanced directive exists unless there is a wallet card indicating where the directive is, who to call about it, or other information about it. To have a choice, the nature of the choice must be shared. Advanced directives of either type do no good if no one knows the document has been made.

When writing the document (or filling in the form) at least two witnesses who are not beneficiaries of the person's estate should sign the directive. Sometimes the nurse is asked to be a witness. Copies should be given to a trusted family member, a doctor or a lawyer, and others told who has the copy in case of need. The document needs to be reviewed and updated on a regular basis to be sure it still reflects what the signer wants to happen. If a family member or friend believes that a person who wrote an advanced directive many years ago has changed desires, and has some testimony by others to that effect, that friend may have the court suspend the directive. Advanced directives should be initialed and dated after review each year to document the current wishes of the person making the directive.

Health care professionals are required to abide by the advanced care directive unless the patient is told beforehand that one or more of the provisions are against the policy of the institution or group. In that case, they must inform the patient in writing, and in case of conflict, follow state law. Sometimes institutions or state offices (e.g., the Governor's office) have ombudsmen who can arbitrate such conflicts. The ombudsman will see that all legal rights are protected. Other people who can help resolve conflict include the hospital administrator, risk management officer, hospital chaplain or other clergy, social worker, and the hospital ethics committee. The ethics committee is composed of a variety of people from several disciplines, including nursing, medicine, theology or philosophy, the community, and sometimes other interested people. They review ethical issues on a case-by-case basis, acting for society in determining all ethical options and facilitating decision making, balancing the needs and rights of all parties.

For the dying person, it is wise to know hospital or hospice or institutional policy as it relates to the advanced directive before being admitted. For example, a hospice may not provide cardiopulmonary resuscitation (CPR) for those who die while hospice personnel are present. That fact is shared with patients before admission to hospice. If a living will specifies that CPR is wanted, that hospice may not be the best choice of care provider. Or a patient may want to have someone in addition to hospice personnel be present during acute episodes to provide CPR. The patient may decide to enter the hospital when death is near, so that CPR will be done. Health care institutions/organizations must record the fact that a patient has made an advanced directive. That record is found on patients' charts.

The widely reported cases of Karen Ann Quinlan and Nancy Cruzan showed the enormous effort it can take families to get the legal system to allow them to discontinue certain life-support measures. In both cases, the young women were diagnosed to be in a persistent vegetative state, or irreversible coma, and needed supportive care to survive. Neither of the young women had made a living will, but families of both women believed that they knew their wishes regarding living the way they were living. The family of Nancy Cruzan wanted to stop the artificial hydration and feeding that was keeping her alive. The family of Karen Ann Quinlan wanted to stop the respirator ventilating her. After Karen Ann Quinlan's ventilator was removed, she lived another nine years. The families were mired in the legal system for years, at tremendous burden, before reaching a satisfactory conclusion. People who know they are dying can spare their families this burden.

The legal principles defined in part because of these two cases include:

- There is a constitutional right of competent adult patients to be free of unwanted medical treatment.

- This right continues even if the patient is subsequently unable to make medical decisions.

- Different states may have different standards to determine if the patients left information that would clearly show their desire to be treated or not to be treated in different circumstances.

- The state has an interest in preserving life.

- The United States Supreme Court recognized the enforceability of advanced directives. (Hill & Shirley, 1992, pp. 5–11)

Not having an advanced directive means not having a choice. End-of-life wishes may not be honored, even if they are known, if they are not recorded. If family or others know what the wishes are, they must find ways to prove them by testimony of people who heard the patient say what was wanted, or find diaries or other written records expressing choice. This requires more time, money, energy, and emotion by loved ones.

CARING FOR THE CAREGIVER

With all the expectations society has for caregivers, the connecting, truth telling, and advocacy as well as the physical, financial, and emotional care, caregiver burnout is a real problem. Supporting family caregivers is as much a part of the multidisciplinary team effort as is care of the dying patient (see Figure 8-1).

All family or friends in the caregiver role should be encouraged to take care of themselves. This is often difficult to do with increasing physical care demands, and the emotional upheaval and need to reassess one's role in life based on the impending loss. Caregivers should be encouraged and supported in doing some very basic things that include:

- recognize physical limitations and get help with lifting, turning, and other physical care
- exercise daily, at least as much as you are used to doing
- sleep as much as needed, and plan sleep around the patient's sleeping habits, if necessary
- eat a balanced diet regularly, and weigh on the same scale three times a week to guard against precipitous or unplanned weight loss
- drink enough water to avoid dehydration; avoid over indulgence in alcohol or caffeinated drinks
- allow others who offer to cook, shop, or do other tasks to do so
- avoid carrying infection by washing hands regularly before and after patient care and moisturizing the skin afterwards
- maintain regular health care, including doctor and dentist visits
- consider respite care, either through home care, respite inpatient care, friends staying with the patient, or adult day care if appropriate (see McFarlane & Bashe, 1998).

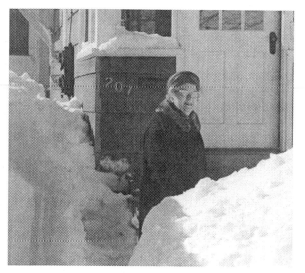

Figure 8-1
This caregiver needed help to shovel the snow from her walk.

One elderly man was the sole caregiver for his invalid wife who was in decline, but would probably live several more months, if not a year. During a home visit by a parish nurse, he disclosed that his doctor wanted him to go right into the hospital for diagnosis and treatment of left chest pain. He refused because he felt he needed to care for his wife. The nurse was able to arrange for inpatient respite care at a nearby nursing home for the wife. Only after he had seen that his wife was in the bed receiving care would he enter the hospital for his own needed care. Ten days later, following coronary artery bypass surgery, he returned to his caregiving role with support from his friends and the community. This man needed the team to support him in his health needs so that he could continue his caregiving role. He would not have gone to the hospital for his own care had they not assisted him with the arrangements for his wife.

Caregivers who are caring for a parent, sibling, or someone other than their spouse may need to attend to their mate. A spouse can feel left out if there are long absences, or if the caregiver returns home tired every day and unable to perform the routine tasks usually attendant on her. Caregiving includes making time for the family members, especially the spouse or significant other. Encourage the caregiver to talk about what is going on, ask for help when needed, and plan special times to go out with each other—just the two of them.

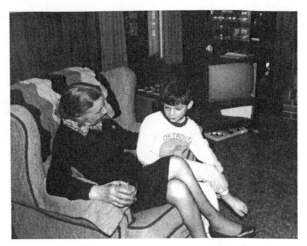

Figure 8-2
Honesty in discussions
with children is vital.

Children in the family also need attention. Age-appropriate discussions about the nature of what is happening helps a child feel included, and that honest answers are forthcoming (see Figure 8-2). The child may feel guilty; may regress and start doing things he did not do recently, like bedwetting; may change behavior, becoming "too good" or aggressive; or may fail in school. Rules of thumb to help children include:

- maintaining a regular schedule
- letting everyone caring for the child, including teachers, babysitters, and others, know what is going on
- involve them in caregiving if they want to be involved
- schedule special time with them
- use counselors with expertise in childhood grief, if necessary
- consider summer camp programs where children who are grieving can share their experiences with other children (like those run by Hospice Organizations)
- help children see they did nothing to cause the crisis

Obviously, caring for the caregiver includes much more than is recorded here. Spiritual health, emotional health, and physical health may all be fragile in this intensely personal and critical time in life. Nurses and others who care for families should assess their needs regularly and consider them as important as patient care. There are many resources for assisting caregivers (see Chapter 9). Use them as appropriate.

SUMMARY

As easy as it sounds, telling the truth, standing up for your patients and their families, and knowing how they can protect their rights are very simple, yet profound, values on which to build a healing relationship. Truth and advocacy are both rooted in the need to have adequate and accurate information in order to make decisions. The right to self-determination is more important than the paternalistic pattern of protecting patients from painful knowledge. That kind of paternalism leads to anxiety, lack of trust, and hopelessness, with people often imagining things to be much worse than they really are. Society has encoded the right to self-determination into law, providing several means by which people can express their preferences in end-of-life issues. These rights should be exercised with consultation with the family. And the family has the right and expectation of having its needs included in the care of family in crisis.

REFERENCES

Chatzky, J. S. (2000). The last word. *Money Magazine, 29*(9), 172.

Donahue, P. (1985). Advocacy. In G. Bulechek & J. McCloskey (Eds.), *Nursing interventions: Treatments for nursing diagnoses*. Philadelphia: W. B. Saunders Co.

Dunn, H. (1994). *Hard choices for loving people*. Herndon, VA: A & A Publishers.

Gadow, S. (1980). An ethical model for assisting patients with treatment decisions. In C. B. Wong & J. Swazey (Eds.), *Dilemmas of dying*. Boston: G. K. Hall Medical Publishers, Inc.

Hill, T. P., & Shirley, D. (1992). *A good death: Taking more control at the end of your life*. Reading, MA: Addison Wesley.

Kübler-Ross, E. (1969). *On death and dying*. New York: McMillan.

Livingston, D., & Williamson, C. (1985). Truth Telling. In G. Bulechek & J. McCloskey (Eds.), *Nursing interventions: Treatments for nursing diagnoses*. Philadelphia: W. B. Saunders Co.

McFarlane, R., & Bashe, P. (1998). *The complete bedside companion*. New York: Simon & Schuster.

Ott, B., & Hardie, T. L. (1997). Readability of advanced directive documents. *Image: Journal of Nursing Scholarship, 29*(1), 53–58.

CHAPTER 9

Resources for the Dying and their Families

THE NEED

Many organizations help people who are dying. Some of their goals are to help dying people

- achieve personal goals at the end of life

- secure care for themselves or family members at home

- grieve after the death of a loved one

- find alternative treatments that complement medical care and help the dying person remain comfortable and at peace.

This chapter focuses on finding those resources. Some are large, national resource groups. Three of these groups are part of the federal government and include the Veterans Administration System, the National Institutes of Health, and Medicare. Hospice is another. A few other large organizations that commonly provide help to dying people are associated with nonprofit voluntary agencies or professional associations. A nurse with a strong professional network and local involvement in a health care community can be creative in using these resources to help a dying person live well until death.

The Internet has become a major resource for finding information and help for people who are dying as well as their families. Web sites provide a means to communicate directly with agencies and organizations

Arthur's Helpers

Arthur, a gay man with Acquired Immune Deficiency Syndrome (AIDS), was having a hard time. His health care was provided by a free clinic, but surgery was required and the local hospital did not want to admit him for the procedure. Surgeons were not willing to operate because they feared the virus. When he did find a county hospital willing to do the surgery, he was very sick, and a prolonged convalescence of at least six weeks was expected. He was discharged in 10 days, unable to care for himself. His prognosis was guarded. He would recover from the surgery, but no one could predict the course of the AIDS.

A coalition of gay men and lesbian women had organized a self-help group to help people like Arthur. They sent members of the group to clean his house, leave two meals a day, keep the lawn mowed, and do the shopping as long as Arthur needed that help. He also had a driver to take him to his follow-up appointments. He recovered, was able to care for himself in about three weeks (except for yard work, which required two months further help), and was relatively well for another year. The provision of simple housekeeping services and food were all that he required.

that provide information at any time of the day or night. In addition, electronic mail can be used to communicate with others who have had similar experiences, a "virtual" support group. Knowledge and skill in the use of the Internet and the ability to teach families to access these sites is an important attribute for nurses.

FINDING RESOURCES

Many people who have a terminal illness need help. Some, like Arthur, live alone but are members of a group who have the resources to assist their members. Others have families or live with people who need basic information on how to help with both physical care and the provision of basic human needs. Some families are unable to provide such help because they are worn out, or are themselves ill. Other families are dysfunctional, barely able to care for members of the family when they are healthy. The impending death immobilizes and paralyzes the family, as discussed previously. The nurse's role in healing the dying becomes one of forging or supporting connections and relationships between the dying patient and groups or individuals willing to help.

Connecting the patient with the resources needed for care requires knowledge of resources and the ability to either recommend them to patients who will use them independently or to make the necessary referrals. A list of useful national resources, both hot lines and addresses of national organizations that have information, publications, referral resources, or specific kinds of assistance available to individuals, can be found in appendix 2, along with the Web site address, if available. Local organizations vary significantly in the type and amount of assistance they offer to individuals.

Nurses can get listings of helpful local groups in several ways. National organizations will refer inquirers to local affiliates. Local libraries often maintain lists (sometimes for sale) of community organizations. These lists are updated annually or bi-annually, usually include phone numbers, and may be categorized into a section on health for easy reference. The League of Women Voters and local chapters of national organizations like the American Red Cross sometimes have lists of agencies that they use for public relations or information. They may charge a small fee for access to the lists. The local health department will have a resource list, possibly on a Web site.

Nurses who work for large institutions or organizations generally have access to people who know about the resources in the geographic area. Case managers, discharge planners, social workers, and even volunteers often know about agencies or groups who provide care, information, or support to dying people. They keep resource lists with current telephone numbers, criteria for enrollment of patients, and costs. They can contact a long list of care providers, including home health agencies, hospice services, home nutrition services, and agencies that provide special services like respiratory care, parenteral nutrition, physical therapy, occupational therapy, homemakers, personal care attendants, financial aid, and respite care. Barriers to using these services include availability, cost, and accurate assessment of need.

One useful way of identifying resources is to remain a part of an organization or network of local nurses who know the resources available and will share that information. Members of specialty organizations often find that one of the most useful benefits of membership is sharing the knowledge of resources others in the group have found. Those resources may include organizations, representatives of companies that give away sample products for testing, alternative care providers, or people with special information who are willing to give educational programs.

One nurse who practiced Therapeutic Touch (TT) in a southeastern state was cited in a national publication. She received a call from a Canadian man concerned about his wife who had been recently diagnosed with breast cancer. He wanted to know how to find a person who practiced TT in Manitoba, and how to go about evaluating alternative health care in general. Because the nurse was a member of the Professional Nurse Healers and had received a directory of practitioners, she was able to refer him to members living close to his hometown who could help him. Directories of nurses and other health care personnel with specialized practices (e.g., diabetes nurse educators) can be very useful.

Patients, too, often find resources that they are entitled to use. Companies they work for may provide benefits. Lodges or groups like the Shriners provide care to children if certain qualifications are met. Religious affiliation may provide access to resources. One church raised $50,000 to help a member get on a heart transplant list, another provided visitors to a man who was dying and needed to talk.

Parish nursing is developing in some areas as a means for churches to address more comprehensive care needs of parishioners. Parish nurses are registered nurses who work, or sometimes volunteer, in faith communities of all kinds. There are currently about 15,000 RNs functioning in this role. They do not replicate services available in the community, and they are not home health nurses. The role is defined as: advocate, educator, counselor (within the legal definition of counseling in each state), referral agent, and coordinator of volunteers. Most parish nurses consider their role a part of the health ministry of the faith community, so they focus on spiritual needs and whole person health, as well as health promotion and wellness in the traditional sense. If a person who is dying is a member of a faith community that has a parish nurse, that nurse is an invaluable resource. A care team may be formed to provide homemaker service, lawn services, babysitting for the family children, and other tasks, all under the direction of the nurse. The parish nurse will work with both the patient's doctor and the family to make appropriate referrals at appropriate times (e.g., to hospice for increased pain control services). Other services depend on the nature of the parish nurse role as defined by the congregation or faith community and the perceived needs of that community.

Use of the Internet

Health care providers must be computer literate, especially in the use of the Internet, to identify and refer those in need to resources, both informational and service providers. Any personal library should include a book or two on how to search for resources online, appropriate listings of relevant Web sites, and links to national resources offered by government and voluntary agencies.

When beginning a search for information or specific resources, if you know an organization or agency web address, go to that Web site directly. For example, you can access the National Library of Medicine directly (www.nlm.nih.gov) and once you are into their web pages, you can follow their advice and directions to search that database. *Consumer Reports* (2000) suggests that for information on a medical topic start with MEDLINE plus, a site that is authoritative, updated regularly, and focused. Read search tips to learn how to narrow the search to a manageable number of citations, limiting the search to review articles or clinical trials, depending on the information needed. Librarians can help you.

If you want to search for information that may be incorporated into several databases, use a search engine. Search engines are tools that quickly scan thousands of Web sites by keyword or other parameter. So, if you were looking for information on vitamin therapy for persons with AIDS, you would use a search engine (e.g., Alta Vista, HotBot, or others). Comparisons of search engines by speed, comprehensiveness of the database, and ease of use are published regularly (McGuire, Stilbourne, McAdams, & Hyatt, 1997). Become familiar with one or two and use them well. Metasearch engines (e.g., Dogpile) search multiple search engines at once. This makes your search more comprehensive, but may result in thousands of citations, or sites, unless you can refine your search to a very specific topic. You may spend a lot of time reading individual Web sites written by lay people who want to share their experiences, rather than current medical information (Nicoll & Ouellette, 1997).

National Organizations usually have Web sites that identify what services and information are offered, the cost, and local links. When visiting these Web sites, be sure to check when they were last updated to determine if the information is current. Note, too, if they give information and links to related sites that are not organizationally related to them.

Local providers often have Web sites. Hospitals, health care organizations, public health agencies, police and fire departments, and local branches of the American Red Cross and other organizations are likely to have local information listed. You can find information similar to the data that case managers of local hospitals have on the local Web sites of these agencies. The local community service organization, public health agency, or other group may have put together an index of resources for the local area, like a directory. This can be a useful tool.

Compassionate care of those who are dying requires the use of multiple resources. Tools to find those resources that are available in any area include knowledgeable people, published sources, and the Internet.

MAKING REFERRALS

Referral to an agency that provides direct care on a fee-for-service basis is probably the easiest and most common approach to providing care for the dying for those who can afford it or who have insurance that covers it. Gaps in referrals and lack of continuity of care between hospital and home can occur for several reasons, with lack of monetary resources comprising only part of the problem.

Persons treated in a large referral hospital may live in a different geographical area, and the staff of the hospital may not know community resources available there. These hospitals generally refer to a primary care service. That service may not be aware of all the needs of the dying individual related to treatments rendered at the referral center. For that reason, careful documentation is a crucial part of the referral process, with a telephone call between discharge nurse and new agency a crucial way to clarify what treatments were given, how care is being done, and what the nurse believes will be needed at the home or place of discharge. If a visit by the home care provider to the patient before discharge from the hospital is possible, it is very useful for planning purposes and for getting any physician's orders needed for medications and treatments. The referral process requires that the discharge nurse has done a careful assessment of the patient and family, both needs and strengths, and has thoughtfully planned for future needs. Networks of providers, including nurses, are continually being created both formally and informally, and they aid the referral process.

Unfortunately, too often the need for services is not apparent while a person is hospitalized or receiving active treatment. Even if the need is assessed appropriately, once the person is discharged and the needs change, a reassessment may not be done. For example, a primary care practitioner following a patient through office visits may not be told of nonmedical problems, like caregiver fatigue or diminishing functional ability with regard to food preparation, and may not ask about it. People with serious needs often do not know where to go for help. Help can be classified as either information services or agencies/people who provide care.

GOVERNMENT

Organizations may be grouped by type of ownership: for profit, government, or not-for-profit organizations. Profit-making services are often included as home health services within a corporation devoted to health care. They can be found in each community, and often reflect the social and economic background of that community. An example is the fact that health food stores may be found in communities with socially sophisticated, upwardly mobile young professionals, while no such options are in evidence in inner city neighborhoods.

Resources for the care of dying people are provided by both the federal government and various state and local governments. Two of the largest federal programs that provide direct services to people are the V.A./military system and the Department of Health and Human Services (HHS). HHS is responsible for the Health Care Financing Agency (HCFA), administrators of the Medicare program, the Social Security Administration, which manages payments for disabled people as well as aged or blind people, and the U.S. Public Health Service, which is responsible for the Agency for Healthcare Research and Quality.

Veterans Administration

The federal government has programs useful for military and retired military personnel who are dying, whether or not the reason for the final illness is service connected. Often found within Veterans Administration Hospitals, services for the dying include both inpatient and outpatient medical care, prescribed drugs and equipment like ostomy supplies, treatments, and financial services. Offices within the Veterans Administration (V.A.) will help veterans determine if they are eligible for care within the V.A. system. Programs of care vary between hospitals, some providing inpatient hospice-like care, others being only acute care facilities. Most will provide needed medication. Veterans' groups often volunteer time and resources for their military compatriots, visiting them and offering toiletries, entertainment, and a sense of belonging to the larger group. In the natural reminiscence that takes place, people resolve many old issues.

Research Information from the Federal Government

The National Institutes of Health (NIH) are supported by the U.S. government for the purpose of research and have a variety of treatment programs underway at all times. Doctors working in the National Cancer Institute (NCI), National Institute of Mental Health (NIMH), Heart

Mr. Bower's Buddies

It was a day Mr. Bower usually tried to forget. Years before, in Korea, his platoon had been fired on, and several of his friends had been wounded. Two of them had died. During the fight, Mr. Bower had distinguished himself (he never said what he did), and was commended for his heroism. On the anniversary of the fight, three of the men who had been there and now lived in Mr. Bower's city showed up at the V.A. hospital and had a ceremony to honor those who had fought. Remembering the two who had died, and being honored for helping the living, Mr. Bower finally came to a peace about that incident in his life. His comrades in arms, through their thoughtfulness to the whole group, helped one dying member to find peace.

Lung and Blood, and others admit patients to rigidly controlled studies. Appropriate patients for research programs are referred by other practicing physicians. People wishing to fight their disease by becoming study subjects should ask their physicians for information, or ask the doctor to call the National Institute of Health that relates to their problem to determine if any of the current studies are appropriate for them. The National Cancer Institute maintains a database called Physicians Data Query, or PDQ, that lists protocols and study information on at least 85 treatments, with 1,000 protocols and 12,000 physicians (Lesko, 1994).

The U.S. government maintains many information services related to health care. An example is the Agency for Healthcare Research and Quality that publishes guidelines for treatment on such topics as pain control, pressure sores, incontinence, depression, and other problems that commonly complicate the care of dying people. Information for patients or clinicians can be obtained without cost (see Table 9-1).

Hot lines are maintained to provide access to information, offer referral services, and sometimes provide financial assistance. Private agencies as well as the government maintain hot lines and Web sites as

TABLE 9-1	Selected Print Resources, Government

Agency for Healthcare Research and Quality

Clinical guidelines relevant to the care of the dying are available from this agency by writing to:

  AHCPR Clearinghouse
  P.O. Box 8547
  Silver Springs, MD 20907

or calling 1-800-358-9295. Guidelines available include:

  Pressure Ulcers in Adults: Prediction and Prevention

  Urinary Incontinence in Adults

  Evaluation and Management of Early HIV Infection

  Acute Pain Management: Operative or Medical Procedures and Trauma

  Management of Cancer Pain: Adults

Social Security Administration

Information about financial assistance available through this agency can be obtained by writing to:

  Department of Health and Human Services
  Social Security Administration
  Baltimore, MD 21235

Booklets available include:

  Understanding Social Security

  Medicare

  Disability

  A Guide to SSI for Groups and Organizations

  Survivors

All of these resources are available without charge.

efficient methods of distributing health care information. The National Health Information Center (P.O. Box 1133, Washington, DC, 20013) can send a publication catalog. Two of the publications cited are a list of selected Federal Health Information Clearinghouses and Information Centers and Toll-free Numbers for Health Information. Appendix 2 lists a few of those that relate to common problems of the dying patient or to certain disease states. Each nurse will want to check the current telephone number of the relevant hot lines in a current directory of 800 numbers or through directory assistance, and keep the information updated in a resource file specific to the case load.

Local Government

State and local governments vary by locale in terms of the provision of care and information that help dying patients. A variety of social programs help to feed and care for people who lack the financial means to help themselves, though programs are limited and often there is not enough to meet all the needs. Food banks, food stamps, Medicaid funds, county hospitals for indigent patients (often supported in part by both state and county), community health clinics (including those for specific diagnoses like AIDS), transportation vouchers for trips to the hospital, and home health aid programs are found in many localities. Each governmental unit has its own set of regulations and requirements for enrollment. Quasi-governmental agencies, those supported in part by the government through grants and other means, like senior citizen centers in some places, may have volunteers and other programs that support dying people, with different requirements for enrollment.

States provide regulation and monitoring of care facilities and care providers for the protection of the public through licensing. There is a mechanism in each state that receives and investigates complaints about substandard care given to patients should a family be concerned. The State Board of Nursing for the state serves that function for complaints about nurses. A national Disciplinary Data Base (DDB) is maintained listing practitioners (including physicians and nurses) who have been disciplined in their states or who have malpractice claims filed against them. If a family or a nurse suspects substandard care is being given to a dying patient in an institution that is licensed, the licensing agency should be notified and asked to investigate. If the institution is not licensed, or the agency is slow to respond, contact the Office of the Governor, the ombudsman for health care. This person will investigate complaints about patient care, questions of abuse, and so on. Standards of Nursing Practice mandate the reporting of substandard care.

NONGOVERNMENTAL ORGANIZATIONS

Voluntary agencies provide support to people who meet their criteria. Because each agency has different criteria that change frequently, the search for support can be confusing and frustrating. That is why consulting with people who do discharge planning or home health is often a useful first step—they have up-to-date information and can save many phone calls and letters. The best-known and most comprehensive set of services offered specifically for dying patients is offered by Hospice, a fee-for-service organization.

Hospice

Hospice is not a place, it is a "well-coordinated set of services intended to relieve or ease the varied symptoms or side effects of a terminal illness" (Beresford, 1993). Hospice staff and volunteers help people live well until they die. The overall goal is to provide comfort and care for people who are dying and their families. It usually occurs in the home or nursing home, but some inpatient hospice units exist.

St. Christopher's in Sydenham, England, is usually considered the first modern hospice. Hospice care first developed when human beings formed settled communities and began to care for sick people. Many had religious orientations, such as those associated with Egyptian, Oriental, Greek, and Roman temples that were used as refuges for travelers and the sick. Christianity and Islam both supported the care of the sick as a religious duty and built peaceful hospice structures throughout their respective territories. Crusaders spread the hospice idea by helping to build hospices on their way to and from crusades and by using them when weary and attempting to return home to England (Siebold, 1992, p. 16). The hospices provided respite and kindness, but not medical care.

During the Dark Ages, many hospices disappeared and others became almshouses, places where disease was not controlled and no one went if they had a choice. When modern medicine developed, hospices became hospitals, devoted to the cure of disease. But a few hospices dedicated to the care of the incurably ill continued or were reborn. In 1879, Our Lady's Hospice opened to provide palliative care for the terminally ill, the first facility created under religious auspices to do so in the nineteenth century. Sister Mary Aikenhead, an Irish nun who had worked with Florence Nightingale and was knowledgeable about the French hospices associated with the order of St. Vincent De Paul, was credited with being the inspiration for the opening of that hospice (Siebold, 1992).

Two women became charismatic and outspoken advocates of the hospice movement in the 1950s and 1960s. Dr. Cicely Saunders developed a comprehensive program of physical, emotional, and spiritual care for palliation of symptoms and support of people who were dying and their families. Dr. Elizabeth Kübler-Ross supported such a movement based on her studies of the process of dying, the identified need for such support, and the obvious benefits to those people and their families when such support was given. Through the efforts of Dr. Saunders, St. Christopher's Hospice in England became a model of care for the dying, a place to demonstrate how to care for people who could not be cured. Through the efforts of Dr. Kübler-Ross, the awareness of the emotional and spiritual needs of terminally ill people was popularized.

It is not possible to move one system of care, like hospice, into a different culture just as it is where it was developed. The English system changes as it is adopted by U.S. care professionals because laws, regulations, and cultural norms are different. Saunders writes of differences between American and British physicians, stating that as a British physician, she was willing to carry out, not write, orders for ancillary staff (Siebold, 1992, p. 71). Hers is an interdisciplinary approach, and the doctor is not always the team leader. In the United States, medical directors of hospice units or organizations are usually physicians and usually consider themselves team leaders. Other times, the medical director works closely with the patient's own physician who remains the primary physician for the patient. Interdisciplinary respect for the talents of each team member leads to sharing the role of team leader depending on patient needs and goals. The Medicare Hospice Benefits plan outlines what hospice care must consist of for payment by Medicare. Hospice services are reimbursed by most insurance policies, and by Medicare for those entitled to it. Benefits covered by Medicare completely or in part include at least:

- on-call services 24 hours a day, 7 days a week

- professional services of physician, nurse, and social worker

- home health aide and homemaker services

- some medical supplies

- some medications (with a co-payment sometimes required)

- some medical equipment

The National Hospice Organization publishes *Hospice Care,* a comprehensive guide to hospice services and referral service that is useful to anyone caring for the dying (Minnesota Hospice Organization, 1998).

Hospice has developed locally according to the goals, values, and resources of the community it serves. A National Hospice Organization serves as a clearinghouse of information, and can refer people to local hospice services. Following is a set of objectives with which most hospices in the United States agree:

- The patient participates in the treatment and maintains independence and control as long as possible.

- The patient and family are a unit of care. When the patient dies, the family may need continued care for a period of time.

- The care team is interdisciplinary.

- Pain management and symptom control are major goals.

- Care is affordable.

Enrollment in a hospice generally requires that a patient's values are similar to the hospice. That means that the patient is seeking comfort-oriented care rather than aggressive treatment aimed at extending life at all costs. In the past, some hospices required the patient to sign DNR (do not resuscitate) directives. The M.D. would sign a do-not-resuscitate order based on the patient's directive prior to enrollment. New laws about living wills and other end-of-life issues (the Patient Self-Determination Act of 1991) make that a questionable legal issue. Some people feel it is not legal or ethical to require a patient to surrender rights (in this case, the right to CPR) in order to receive the kind of care otherwise desired.

Enrollment into hospice is fully explained and patient and family, and all consent in writing to hospice care. Referral to hospice services is made by the patient's physician.

Other criteria for enrollment into hospice are:

- Medical diagnosis of a terminal disease, with a prognosis of six months to a year (Medicare requirements are more specific, and change from time to time).

- There must be a caregiver available, usually a family member or significant person in the patient's life, though sometimes a church or organization may take responsibility for caring for a member.

- Hospice care must be provided in a safe setting: safe for patient, family, and hospice worker.

The interdisciplinary team members of a hospice unit assigned to one patient depend on the needs of the individual (see Figure 9-1). Teams meet regularly to develop, maintain, review, and carry out a plan

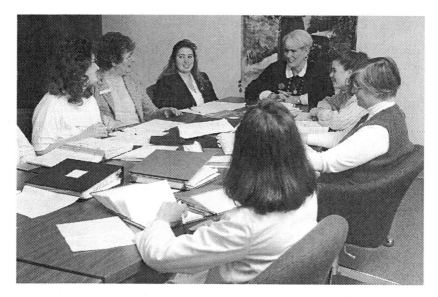

Figure 9-1 The members of the interdisciplinary team will vary depending on the needs of the client.

of care and treatment for the patient. The team works together to achieve consensus on the plan of care so that each team member is committed to the same goals. They organize themselves to visit the patient on different days so that the patient is seen as often as possible. They are careful to document all care for communication as well as for legal reasons.

A typical early arrangement might be for the nurse-case manager to see the patient for evaluation initially and once a week; a care attendant to provide personal care three times a week; and a physical therapist to teach the family safe ways of exercising the patient on an alternate day. The patient or family can call these team members any time, usually asking the nurse to coordinate the calls. The patient's physician, fully a member of the team, follows the patient through office visits and by phone with the registered nurse when the patient's condition changes and new orders are needed.

Volunteers are also members of the team, even if they give most of their time in the hospice office. When they are assigned to a family, they may be used to sit with the patient and give caregivers a few hours off, or they may provide transportation to the doctor's office or other treatment center. They may also walk the dog, deliver medicines, or baby-sit. Most often, they make the family situation easier to manage.

An integral part of the team, the social worker focuses on the financial environment and relationships. Some functions overlap those of the nurse, and if the social worker and the nurse work well together, the overlapping competencies can be a strength of the team. For example, sometimes both the nurse and the social worker are qualified to do supportive counseling. The hospice chaplain may also be qualified to do counseling. In this case, the team will decide who takes on the responsibility for this task based on the relationship with the family and other responsibilities. Other responsibilities of the social worker are listed in Table 9-2, and of the registered nurse in Table 9-3.

Bereavement services are a part of hospice. Bereavement support is available for 13 months following the patient's death in most hospice organizations. People who have worked together to ease the death of another, families and hospice team together, have an intense emotional experience. Meetings at annual candlelight remembrances or other planned events are helpful to both groups of people—just to see how

TABLE 9-2	Hospice Social Worker Responsibilities

Help families get financial services to which they are entitled; for example:
- Medicare
- Medicaid
- Social Security
- Food stamps
- Insurance payments
- Company benefits

Help families with legal issues, such as:
- How to get a will made
- Information on advanced directives, living wills
- Informed consent

Referrals for community services, such as:
- Funeral homes
- Local branches of organizations that can provide equipment like wheelchairs or hospital beds, flags for coffins, and other anticipated needs

Family conferences to resolve conflict, and other types of supportive counseling in collaboration with other team members who are able to offer counseling services.

they are doing. Children, in particular, are cared for in groups or sometimes summer camps, so that they can meet and discuss loss of a loved one with other children in a nurturing environment.

Other Organizations

The American Cancer Society maintains a room across the street from a large medical facility for adult cancer patients who come from out of town for cancer treatments. Nearby, the Ronald McDonald House may be used by children and their families for the same purpose. It is supported by private and corporate funds in many cities. A funeral home offers the services of a Master's degreed bereavement counselor for a month following the death of a loved one as a natural part of the care

TABLE 9-3	Registered Nurse Responsibilities

Coordinates care
- Skilled assessment of patient and family
- Communication with physician
- Communication with other team members
- Follows up with documentation
- Calls team meetings, generally leads them

Provides direct patient care
- Pain control
- Psychological support
- Skilled nursing care requirements
- On-call coverage for crises and to be with patient and family at the time of patient's death
- Family grief counseling after the patient's death

Education
- Patient
- Family
- Care team

they give to clients. The counselor provides group sessions to help family members talk about their loss and move through the immediate period of bereavement. These are examples of private and corporate recognition and funding of resources useful to dying people in one American city.

Hospice services have a clear and coherent set of purposes and guidelines, though local groups vary in some procedural and funding issues. Other organizations are formed around other parameters of care, most often a disease (like cancer), a system (like the heart or kidney or liver), a procedure (like transplantation), or a symptom (like pain). National organizations exist to address many of these problems. If a patient who is dying has needs that are unfulfilled and the family seems unable to meet them, community outreach from these groups is often a viable alternative. Communities exist to care for their members. Creative nurses look for resources for patients from them, if not directly, then through social service workers or volunteers in the agency where the nurse works. As with the funeral director who initiated bereavement counseling for clients, other entrepreneurs in the community are becoming health conscious and willing to offer increasing levels of services. These businesspeople need only to be asked by consumers of their services or products for help that they can give.

SUMMARY

Meeting the needs of dying patients and their families is a part of healing the dying. A caring professional expertly brings to their care the things people need to be able to maintain their quality of life and achieve a sense of peace and continuity of life through family and community. The resources needed vary greatly, taking the form of financial and physical resources like food, equipment, and money, together with people who have knowledge and ability to help with grief and bereavement.

The U.S. government provides major resources in the form of veterans' care, Medicare for aged and disabled citizens, and research plans and care for those who qualify. Large national organizations provide information and more limited access to care, equipment, and services. Hospice services are available in most areas for people who are dying and wish to focus on palliative care. Appendix 2 lists hot lines and resource clearinghouses that may be useful to those seeking resources. Networking with health care professionals who have knowledge of resources in a community is the most effective way to learn of resources.

REFERENCES

Beresford, L. (1993). *The hospice handbook: A complete guide.* Boston: Little, Brown & Co.
Consumer Reports on Health (vol. 12, 2000). *How to research a medical topic on line.* Yonkers, NY: Consumers Union of U.S., Inc.
Lesko, M. (1994). *Lesko's info-power* (2nd ed.). Detroit, MI: Visible Ink Press.

Mcguire, M., Stilbourne, L., McAdams, M., & Hyatt, L. (1997). *Internet handbook for writers, researchers, and journalists.* New York: Guilford Press.

Minnesota Hospice Organization (1998). *Hospice care: A physician's guide.* Raleigh, NC: Hospice for the Carolinas.

Nicoll, L. H., & Ouellette, T. H. (1997). *Nurses' guide to the Internet.* Philadelphia: Lippincott.

Siebold, C. (1992). *The hospice movement: Easing death's pains.* New York: Twayne Publishers.

PART IV

Special Cases

CHAPTER 10

Unique Challenges

FAMILY

Nurses care for people who, in their dying, present special problems or have special needs. Some of those problems may belong to the nurse when the patient is someone close, like a parent, spouse, child, or friend. Sometimes those patients have a stigmatizing illness, like Acquired Immune Deficiency Syndrome (AIDS). Sometimes the patients are victims of violence, like homicide or suicide, and the nurse is concerned with perceived injustice in the world. Sometimes the death is that of a colleague. When death occurs to these people, there are often special considerations in their care and in care for the caregivers.

Death of Parents of Adult Children

The death of a parent is often difficult and complicated because of the history of relationship, and the fact that the loss extends beyond the loss of an individual. For some people, the relationship with the parent is the most stable relationship in life, the place where they can always turn for unconditional love. For others, the relationship has been confusing.

Although it is generally accepted that in the natural order of events parents die before their children, there is always a sense of loss that transcends the death of one person. There is the loss of opportunity to respond, to tell the parent of one's love, and to thank the parent for the many small things given or shared. There is the loss of the opportunity to share significant secrets of life. One man regretted that he had never shared the fact that he was gay with his father and would never know how his father would have reacted to that fact. He continually built fantasies about how he thought his father would have felt, sometimes thinking that the father would have been supportive and loving, other times believing the father would have rejected him. There was no way to confirm either scenario after the death of the father. Somehow the relationship was never complete because the secrets were never shared (Akner, 1993).

For one daughter, the death of a mother meant she lost contact with relatives in Sweden because she had never learned the language. The loss of family ties in the old country was significant to her. Some adult children believe they have never measured up to a parent's standards, and now will never be able to prove themselves. Or they feel guilty for things left undone. For children who have no siblings and are unmarried, the death of a parent may be the death of the whole family. Even adult children may feel abandoned, especially if parent and child never talked about death.

Some children have accepted the caregiving role for their parents for years. The death of a parent who has been the focus of a person's attentions for several years may leave that person feeling less needed by others. It also leaves a hole in the daily schedule, and a need to make choices about what to do with time, how to form new relationships, and decisions about a person's responsibility to others. A person's meaning in life may have been bound to her caretaking activities, and without that responsibility, life loses its meaning.

In the time preceding the death of a parent, hard decisions may have been made. Treatment decisions, such as discontinuing noxious medications, placing parents in care institutions, withdrawing life-support systems, or using needed family resources for care when cure seems hopeless may all burden the family grieving the loss of a parent. If the parent has left explicit instructions for these decisions, it may be easier for the adult children.

When parents die, there is always a change in family relationships. If the family has been dysfunctional, it may have been one parent who kept the peace. If so, someone else must take on that role if the family is to have peace. Or the relationships will need to be repatterned so there is no need for a peacemaker. That is unlikely to happen without help. A mature, functioning family will grieve together, find ways to grow closer, and realign roles.

There are several things that a nurse can do to help adult children who have lost a parent. The first is to realize that the loss is always significant. There is no such thing as finding solace in words like, "He was 95 years old and led a long and healthy life. This was a good way to go." A child of 70 years of age who had a parent for all of those 70 years will be confronted with mortality and feel alone. There will be a need for a period of grieving and then a connection with others for healing to occur. Silence, allowing tears, giving time for the person to remain with a body if necessary to say good-bye, a caring touch on the shoulder, or holding a person's hand all reflect a caring presence and a genuine desire to share the loss. Sharing last words the child may not have heard or a funny story that the parent shared with the nurse about a family member may be a good connection.

An adult who has lost a parent needs to identify the extent of the losses in his life and how to deal with those losses. Support groups for adults who have lost parents are often effective, usually lasting four to six weeks, and help people through some of the intense grief and issues of their own mortality. Clergy, counselors who understand bereavement issues, and family members who are coping well may be excellent resources for follow-up. If depression follows prolonged grieving, professional help is recommended. The nurse who maintains an ongoing relationship with the family, perhaps through hospice or other follow-up services of the organization, should be alert for signs of prolonged grieving, depression, or suicide.

Parents who have prepared well, discussed death with the children, and were able to meet the criteria for a "good death" (e.g., dying alert and without pain, in comfort and having completed the tasks of saying good-bye and accomplishing goals), leave a model of how to die well. If they have prepared financially, left final directives, and shown their children how they fit into the intergenerational family (their place in the interconnectedness of people through the generations), they help the children see death as personally less fearsome, a normal part of life. But they cannot take away the sense of loss and separation. That is a part of love.

Death of Parents of Younger Children

Children who are not adults and lose their parent or parents have a different set of reactions and needs. Not only do they suffer the trauma of separation and loss for a loved one, but there is a "serious developmental interference" (Buckingham, 1990). Their security is threatened. They do not know how to act or what to do when the parent is not there to do the things the child has come to trust that the parent will do. As one small child said when informed of a death, "She never did that before."

Children are unable to grieve intensely for long periods of time, so they have short periods of intense grief and crying, punctuated by periods of watching TV, playing, and doing other things that the adults around them may feel are inappropriate. Yet, the periods that appear to be denial are probably protective, giving the child time to think through this new event. Many children regress in their behavior, moving to a previous stage of development. Bed-wetting may recur after a death in a child who had not been wetting the bed for some time. The child may revert to former speech patterns or thumb sucking or other regressive behavior. Like the crying and the TV watching, this is intermittent.

Grieving children often feel guilty, as if they did something to contribute to the death. They need:

- reassurance that they did not cause the death
- the opportunity and encouragement to express their fears and anger
- to be loved and secure
- to accept their own feelings, alien though they may seem

For them, getting on with their lives means continuing to achieve the appropriate developmental tasks for their ages, including a revised understanding of security.

There are two tasks involved in children's grief. Children must release the sad feelings and accept the loss of the parent (Buckingham, 1990, p. 36). Families are the ideal resource for grieving children, to help with both tasks. However, with the loss of a parent, the whole family is grieving and often finds coping difficult. They can get help from support groups like Hospice, which has a number of programs for grieving children to help them express their feelings via drawings, talking with other children, and sending letters to heaven. Nurses are often active in children's support groups, helping children learn to cope with the loss of a parent. Children's hospitals sometimes have children's support groups, which are run by volunteers, nurses, or sometimes social workers.

Grieving children should always be told the truth in an age-appropriate way. Daddy has not just gone away. If he is dead, he is not coming back, and the child should be allowed to grieve that fact. Otherwise, the sense of abandonment and mistrust is hard to overcome, even later in life. If the child has been with a dying patient, seen the body, talked with others about the impending death as the child is able to understand, the grieving will probably be shorter. The child has been able to begin anticipatory grieving. The child will learn to cope more quickly. The child may have been able to say good-bye. For a child to learn to cope with the death of a loved one, a healing relationship with other family members or caregivers is very important.

Death of a Child

When a child dies, it somehow seems so much worse than when a parent dies. The life seems too short, too unrealized. A wise pediatric nurse said to a weeping student nurse who had lost a three-year-old patient, "Every life, no matter how short, is a complete life." This nurse measured life in something other than time.

The dying child has the same needs for healing relationships as any dying person, and needs for comfort, pain control, reassurance, and care. The child may have gone through many remissions, repeated hospitalizations, varied treatment protocols, and periods of feeling well alternating with periods of feeling very unwell. Such a child is able to play with friends and achieve the developmental progress expected some of the time, but not at other times. If the repeated treatment cycles leave the child with less and less energy, a kind of lethargy and perhaps depression are likely. The child is likely to accept the fact of impending death before the parents do, and sometimes feels guilty about that. It is as if the child wants to get it over with, and get on to the next phase of existence (Buckingham, 1990).

Most people who work with dying children know that honesty is the basis of trust, and there is really no question about telling the child that death is probable. The child will know and will ask quite directly if she is going to die, but only if she feels she will get an honest answer and that her question will not hurt the one she asks too much. Asking a parent may not be possible if the child is aware the parent is avoiding the subject and cannot deal with it. The child may ask someone else, like a nurse. When working with a dying child, the nurse should be prepared when the child says something like, "I know I'm going to die." Reflexively denying the possibility is not helpful to the child. Admitting that death is a possibility opens the door to future discussion. The child's questioning should indicate how much and when information should be given. The child may initially be seeking specific information about how much pain is likely or whether a family pet will be present in heaven. Encouraging the child to draw pictures and share the drawings can be helpful. The pictures will often include scenes of the afterlife from the child's point of view. The child can role-play games about death with dolls to work out feelings, and discuss death with understanding people—other children, teachers, and the family.

If the nurse does discuss death with a child, the family should know that the child is able to discuss the topic. When the family members are able to handle the conversation, they can be helped to share their understanding with the child in conversation. Past experience with death in the family is a building block that can help the family get more direct with each other and with the child about the child's feelings about her own impending death. Although it is important to be honest and direct with children to the extent that they seem to want to talk, it is important to realize that as with adults, there is always hope. Neither life nor the time of death is ever certain. The hope may be for a quick end, more time, less pain, or many other things. Children have spiritual needs just as adults do, and often find prayer or meditation comforting and satisfying, especially if it has been a routine in the home.

Some older children find meaning in their illness, and a way to fight the illness by discussing it directly with others. Teens share their experiences with peers at camps during the summer or in treatment facilities as they can. Ryan White, a teen dying from AIDS contracted through blood transfusions, was well-known for fighting the injustice of social isolation up to the time of his death. When the school board refused to let him attend school, fearing infection of healthy children, he not only sued the board to allow him to pursue his education, but spoke publicly to lawmakers, other children, and the news media to educate them on the facts of transmission of HIV and how it feels to be dying. He even wrote a book on his experiences (White & Cunningham, 1991). Teens might find it helpful to read his book and know that others have feelings about death that may be quite similar to their own.

Children worry about leaving parents in grief. Some people think that worry can prolong the struggle and preclude a peaceful death. One loving family had a six-year-old son who battled with leukemia for three years. On his last day, he told his mother he didn't want her to be sad, and she would be sad when he died. Later in the day, he began to bleed, and his respirations were agonal. But it seemed he was still struggling for every breath. His mother whispered to him that it might be time for him to let go, and if it was, she wanted him to know that she would always love him, but she and his father would be all right. He immediately stopped struggling, soon slipped into unconsciousness, and peacefully died two hours later. This mother did not hasten the child's death, but she may have made it more comfortable.

Helping parents through the death of a child requires compassion and tolerance. If the death was expected, the family may have discussed such issues as organ donation prior to the death. If it was sudden, as in the case of an accident, they will be asked to make important decisions about organ donation, choice of mortuary or funeral home, and other things they may never have thought about with regard to their child. They will be asked to make these decisions during a time of shock. Parents will probably need some time with the child, to be allowed to hold him, and the nurse must be sensitive to their need for support or privacy. They may need family, counselors, or other significant people in their lives, perhaps their own parents. If no one is available, the nurse may call the hospital chaplain, social worker, hospice bereavement counselor, or other person who can help with support and decision making.

Sudden Infant Death Syndrome (SIDS)

SIDS is a special problem because in most societies, parents are supposed to protect and care for their infants. For most SIDS deaths, defined as the sudden death of an infant who previously appeared healthy, there was no warning of impending death, no way the parents could have known the child needed protection or care. But the parents will experience intense grief, anger, fear, and guilt. Many parents imagine that others look at them with judgment, wondering how they could have let their child die.

The beginning of healing for these parents is the closure of their current relationship with the infant. After the child has been pronounced dead, the parents need to hold the child, sometimes several times between the death and the funeral. Health care workers are urged to treat the infant's body as a child, keeping it swaddled in a blanket, and holding it like a baby. Leaving it unclothed and unattended on a stretcher or in the back of a mortuary vehicle can be extremely upsetting to parents who continue to be parents and see the infant as needing care and protection (Corr, Fuller, Barnickol, & Corr, 1991). Parents need to have respectful attention, privacy when requested, and a place to express emotion. Some specific things that can be offered are:

- allowing them to take something of the infant's, like a lock of hair or the baby blanket

- offering to arrange transportation home from the emergency room or to call family members

- keeping them fully informed, including who to call about autopsy results

- making referrals, including the local SIDS network

These parents in particular will be cut off from other parents with young children, and afraid for their other children, existing or planned. They need connection with family and those who understand SIDS. And they need information about subsequent risk of SIDS for other children.

Siblings

The death of a child may have profound effects on siblings. Through the course of a long illness, siblings may have received less attention than the sick child and have strong feelings about perceived lack of love or parental favoritism for the ill child. They may have felt less important than the dying child, even rejected. When that child dies, the sibling often feels guilty, as if negative thoughts or jealously caused the death. The sibling may have lost a good friend, if a close relationship existed with the sick child. The sibling who does not understand the nature of illness may also feel that she will die.

Helping the siblings is much like helping a child understand the death of a parent. They need to be able to express feelings, and ultimately move on in life to achieve their own developmental tasks. Parents should be encouraged and reminded to help these children by talking with them. Appropriate goals are to help them get back into a stable routine, including school or other regular daily activity, and to understand short-term regressive behavior, like fear of the dark, that may be exhibited following the death. Children's support groups, school counselors, and mental health experts are all potential resources for the child who continues to have difficulty.

Death of a Spouse

The death of a spouse, like the death of a parent or the death of a child, is always unique and seems devastating. Two human beings have chosen to create a life together that no one else could have created. When one is left, the life is different, often significantly so. How a surviving spouse copes depends on the nature of the life created together, the nature of the death, and the environment. Factors associated with spouses who do not move through the grief and continue to have difficulty for a prolonged time include:

- sudden untimely death of the spouse
- multiple losses

- high dependency on the deceased

- perceived lack of support

- poor health prior to bereavement (Benoliel, 1991)

A nursing responsibility is to identify these risk factors and to act to lessen the effects. For example, in Chapter 3, Mrs. J. lost her husband, and only a few months later chose to have heart surgery. She had been coping with her poor health prior to bereavement. Her decision was supported by the nurse.

People who have created a life together in which there is a mutual dependency will each have deficits when living life alone. For example, an aging wife who depended on her husband to drive will have transportation problems to solve. A young husband who does not know how to feed a young child may need to learn to warm a bottle. If one spouse handled all the family finances and dies first, the other will need to learn about money—where it is, how much there is, and how to get it. These secondary losses are significant. Referral to social workers may be helpful or family financial planners, if available.

In the time immediately after the death, the communication skill of listening helps to identify the importance of ideas such as, "What will I do now?" It is important to realize that the person may not be asking for direction concerning who to call or what other immediate actions are necessary. The person may be asking, "What do I do with the rest of my life?" Focusing on the immediate problems may be a way to avoid thinking about long-term changes for a while, but it may also be necessary. The skillful nurse or counselor knows when to assist the grieving spouse to move forward. A discussion of helping all people through grief is found in Chapter 3. The surviving spouse will redefine the meaning of an individual life, perhaps seek meaning in death, and create a new life without the spouse.

STIGMATIZING ILLNESS

Stigmatization by society is the characterization of some diseases or problems as a disgrace, in some way bad or morally reprehensible. It leads to people who have those problems becoming isolated, lonely, unsupported, and often starts a downward spiral toward decreasing health. Examples are the stigmatization of Acquired Immune Deficiency Syndrome (AIDS), violence, or suicide. AIDS, in particular, is the stigmatizing disease of the 1990s, as tuberculosis was earlier in the century.

Acquired Immune Deficiency Syndrome (AIDS)

The stigmatization that comes from having AIDS is due to the fact that the first identified groups of People With AIDS (PWAs) were members of socially disenfranchised minority groups (like poor Haitians), or engaged in socially unacceptable behavior: intravenous drug users or gay men. Though AIDS strikes heterosexual people, people from any country, and people without high-risk behavior, it continues to be stigmatizing and isolating because it is viewed as incurable and contagious. In some countries in Africa where the HIV infection rate is very high, patients are often not told of their diagnosis. People are afraid of AIDS.

AIDS is not as contagious as once thought. If a person is not engaging in high-risk behavior, even working with AIDS patients on a daily basis poses very little risk, almost none if universal precautions as established by the Centers for Disease Control are always used. High-risk groups include anyone who has sex with another person other than in the context of a monogamous relationship (by both partners), receives unscreened blood products, shares contaminated needles, or is infected through skin breaks by contaminated blood or body fluids. There are a few cases of AIDS on record in which the person seems to have recovered. Although this number is small, it does suggest that even AIDS is not hopeless. AIDS is becoming a chronic illness.

People with AIDS, regardless of how they contracted the disease, often feel guilty, lonely, and alienated, and suffer from poor self-esteem. Some of these feelings are supported by a society that limits access to school for children who have AIDS, argues about mandatory HIV testing, and wants health care workers to be prohibited from caring for the public if the worker is HIV positive. The message society sends is that people with AIDS have fewer rights than the rest of society, are less worthy than others, and are "bad" people.

There is a dynamic tension between some parts of the HIV positive community, particularly the gay and lesbian groups, and other parts of society. The gay community has chosen to become politically active, working for civil rights of people with AIDS and increased research monies to find a cure for AIDS. This activism sometimes clashes with the conservative political values of others and each side offends the other. Healing in the gay community, including those with AIDS, requires dialogue within society. Moffat (1986) discusses a scene she witnessed between a gay man and a mother of an AIDS patient. The mother was trying to change her lifelong stereotypical view of gay people by attending a support group, listening to what was said, and sharing the pain of watching a son suffer. One young man in the group immediately assumed she must have been a bad mother, and told her she should be happy her son had people like himself to love him. This kind of polarization of viewpoints, blaming and judgmental behavior does not help create relationship. It makes healing more difficult and disenfranchises grief.

Self-righteousness by members of groups who feel morally superior to AIDS patients reinforces the patients' poor self-esteem and belief that they should withdraw from others. A new age thinker may convey the idea that wrong thoughts cause or at least support illness. Because the new ager does not have the disease, and the patient does, the message conveyed is one of "I'm better than you because I think right thoughts." Groups who promote the belief that AIDS (and other illnesses) are punishment from God also judge the patient, conveying the message that the person with the disease is bad. It must be remembered by health care professionals that many people who have no high-risk behaviors contract AIDS. To engage in thinking that suggests that those who do engage in high-risk behavior deserve the disease is to be judgmental and will interfere with any ability to establish and maintain a healing environment.

People with AIDS may blame themselves, parents, partners, society, or their God figure for their disease. They need to experience forgiveness for their own guilt, and learn to forgive those others they feel contribute to their problems. They need to develop a connectedness with family and people who support and love them unconditionally.

One of the characteristics of people who survive for a long time with AIDS is the sense of taking control of their lives. They refuse to be thought of as victims. They shop for a doctor who will give them the information they need without requiring treatments they do not want. They use anything they think will help: homeopathic remedies, laughter, vitamins, imagery, faith, hope, optimism, Healing Touch and massage, a balanced diet, exercise, sufficient rest, positive prayer, and love. The nurse can help these people to create an environment in which they can thrive. Requirements for such an environment include:

- an intention to create a place of peace and healing

- people in the environment who are able to connect with those who may have a limited life span

- resources to assist in a search for meaning in life, including counselors, spiritual guides, literature on topics like meditation and retreat centers, and the willingness to talk

- willingness to turn inward, to examine self and identify one's strengths and resources

- creativity—murals on the walls that people can add to with colors or pencils, humor carts, and so on

- plans for notification of sexual partners

Natural History

There is a natural history, a regular pattern to HIV infections, with some group and individual variations, according to the expert panel of the Agency for Health Care Policy and Research (El-Sadr, Oleske, & Agins, 1994). Infection occurs through blood or body fluids (sexual contact and blood transmission via dirty needles or contaminated blood products are the most obvious and common methods). There may be a stage of flu-like symptoms, followed by a period of seropositivity, but no symptoms. The symptomatic stage may occur as long as 10–14 years after the seropositive results are first known. This early stage may last several years before the advanced state of AIDS is experienced (Bouman, 1994). Thus, the person with AIDS may have had many years of living with positive HIV test results, and may have developed many skills and a lot of knowledge about the disease.

Long-term survivors of AIDS do not consider themselves victims. They take charge of their own healing. They have T4/CD4 counts monitored every six months while they are asymptomatic, and they understand that counts above 600 do not bring a recommendation for medication from the established medical community because there is no indisputable evidence that medication helps at this stage. There are so many side effects from the medications available that the physicians usually prefer to wait until a stage at which the medication has been shown to be effective. These survivors also know that T4/CD4 counts less than 500 indicate that antiretroviral therapy should be started, and counts should be monitored more often. Counts under 200 mean that prophylaxis for pneumocystic pneumonia should be started. Long-term survivors generally get the monitoring done, but they follow the medication recommendations selectively, depending on the current knowledge of the AIDS community.

Many HIV positive people continually balance the information they receive from the medical establishment, the popular culture represented by online AIDS information services, health food stores and homeopathic practitioners, and the way they feel intuitively. The nurse should seek knowledge of current AIDS treatments and what AIDS patients, including those who are thought to be terminal within the next year, are doing for themselves. Self-treatment that is complementary to medical care will become a part of the treatment plan the nurse and patient establish together.

Caregivers and HIV infected people know that there is an explosion of knowledge about HIV/AIDS treatments in part due to increased research efforts. Previously published data using T4/CD4 counts alone as indicators are no longer tenable. The ability to measure viral load (HIV RNA) has changed the management of AIDS. Continually reassessing and updating standards of care is critical. New combinations of drugs, including the addition of Protease Inhibitors, improve survival time for many people.

Criteria used by hospice organizations to determine those who probably have an expected life span of six months or less have been published to help organizations determine who should be admitted to hospice care. They are adapted here in Table 10-1.

TABLE 10-1	**Factors Associated with Expected Mortality of Less than Six Months**
CD4	• less than 25 cells/mcL and no acute illness • 50 or more cells/mcL and coexisting non-HIV-related life threatening illness
Viral Load	• HIV RNA greater than 100,000 • HIV RNA less than 100,000 with complications or the decision to forego antiretroviral and prophylactic medications

Associated Complications: HIV related

- CNS lymphoma
- Progressive multifocal leukoencephalopathy
- MAC bacteremia, untreated
- Visceral Kaposi's sarcoma, unresponsive to therapy
- Advanced AIDS dementia complex
- Cryptosporidiosis
- Wasting
- Toxoplasmosis
- Renal failure, no dialysis

Associated Complications: non-HIV related

- Chronic persistent diarrhea for one year
- Persistent serum albumin greater than 2.5 gm/dl
- Concomitant substance abuse
- Age greater than 50
- Decisions to forego antiretroviral, chemotherapeutic, and prophylactic drug therapy specifically related to HIV disease
- Congestive heart failure, symptomatic at rest

Source: *Hospice care: A physicians guide,* 1998.

Special problems that require assessment or screening by the nurse for people who are seriously ill with AIDS include:

1. respiratory conditions, which could indicate pneumocystic pneumonia or tuberculosis, two of the most common opportunistic HIV-related infections

2. oral lesions suggestive of herpes simplex, destructive periodontal disease, and other infections

3. eye problems, the most common of which is cytomegalovirus retinitis (CMV), which results in visual disturbances and vision loss

4. signs of sexually transmitted diseases, including neurosyphilis

5. Pap smears for women to detect invasive cervical cancer (El-Sadr, Oleske, & Agins, 1994)

More information about the care of patients with these conditions and the screening techniques and programs can be found in the AHCPR guidelines (El-Sadr, Oleske, & Agins, 1994).

Death due to AIDS is a different path than most deaths because of the nature of the disease. Dementias may occur, making the patient difficult to deal with, and sometimes dangerous, as was the patient who crouched in a corner and threatened to stick the nurses with his I.V. needle if they approached. Medication to restrain patients who develop combativeness due to dementia and sufficient help for the threatened staff, family, and others must be available. Safety, so that the patient does not unintentionally inflict harm to self or others, becomes an important consideration.

Other serious problems at the time of death for the AIDS patient include difficulty with pain control, skin breakdown because of severe wasting and weight loss, nutritional problems due to poor appetite and oral lesions, and fatigue and weakness. These problems are amenable to careful, planned, and adequate nursing care. If the nurse and those who are significant in the life of an AIDS patient have created a nonstigmatizing environment in which the physical care is combined with sensitive and compassionate concern for the relationships that exist, allowing for forgiveness, choice in the patient's treatment plan, release of anger, and love, the patient will live well until death.

VIOLENT DEATH

Death by one's own hand or the hand and intention of another touches friends, family, and the wider community in a unique way. Suicide and homicide are among the leading causes of death in adolescents. Both leave survivors who have difficulty in understanding why such a thing could have occurred and if something should have been done to prevent it. Survivors are often guilt ridden, though nurses should not assume that guilt is always characteristic.

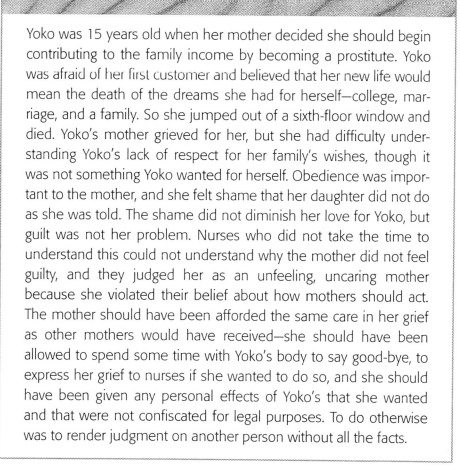

Yoko

Yoko was 15 years old when her mother decided she should begin contributing to the family income by becoming a prostitute. Yoko was afraid of her first customer and believed that her new life would mean the death of the dreams she had for herself—college, marriage, and a family. So she jumped out of a sixth-floor window and died. Yoko's mother grieved for her, but she had difficulty understanding Yoko's lack of respect for her family's wishes, though it was not something Yoko wanted for herself. Obedience was important to the mother, and she felt shame that her daughter did not do as she was told. The shame did not diminish her love for Yoko, but guilt was not her problem. Nurses who did not take the time to understand this could not understand why the mother did not feel guilty, and they judged her as an unfeeling, uncaring mother because she violated their belief about how mothers should act. The mother should have been afforded the same care in her grief as other mothers would have received—she should have been allowed to spend some time with Yoko's body to say good-bye, to express her grief to nurses if she wanted to do so, and she should have been given any personal effects of Yoko's that she wanted and that were not confiscated for legal purposes. To do otherwise was to render judgment on another person without all the facts.

Healing the dying, when the dying occurred unexpectedly as a result of suicide or homicide, requires helping to bridge the chasm that opens between the one who dies and the ones left behind. There has been no opportunity to prepare, to examine existential concerns or meaning in life and death. There may be multiple legal, financial, or social problems. The nurse may meet these survivors in many settings, as stress-related illnesses following this kind of family trauma are not uncommon.

Suicide

Suicide has been called "the cruelest death" (Lester, 1993). People grieving the death of someone whom they feel had a choice to live or die, feel betrayed, angry, puzzled, abandoned, rejected, ambivalent, and strange (Robinson, 1989). Family members may get little support from others, and sometimes ask for none, believing that the dead loved one forfeited a right to the kind of mourning that goes on for others. Religious ritual may be affected by the way the person dies because some groups believe that suicide is a reason to deny burial in consecrated ground. This leads to isolation of the family from the support of that religious organization.

Parents sometimes become overprotective of other children if one child has committed suicide. Some children respond by engaging in risky behavior or losing self-esteem because they obviously can not replace the brother or sister who died and make the parents grieve less. They often feel guilty, believing that if they had fought less, been kinder, or acted differently, the sibling would be alive. They may have trouble understanding that the dead sibling is really dead. Nightmares, poor school work, and depression may follow. Parents may be unaware of these changes because of their own grief.

Friends of teens who commit suicide may be at risk for cluster or copycat suicides. Teens who have already lost a friend to suicide see dying together as glamorous and attention getting. Although rare, it occurs often enough for schools to bring in special counselors when a teen commits suicide to prevent the tragedy of more teens following the pattern. Study of the Bergenfield tragedy, a cluster of four suicides by teens in one carbon monoxide-filled garage, showed that each of the four teens had problems previously (Dolce, 1992). Studies of other clusters confirm that teens do not commit suicide without thought, but suicide by a class-mate or acquaintance may give them the idea of a glamorous way to solve some of their problems. Preventing suicide in this group depends on identifying troubled youths.

If a family has a history of problems, the nurse may make referrals to people who can monitor signs of risk of suicide. These signs include:

- suicide threats
- suicide plans
- previous suicide attempts
- statements about wanting to die
- getting affairs in order
- giving personal treasures away
- personality changes that seem greater than the situation warrants
- withdrawal, apathy, lack of appetite, or other signs of depression
- attempts to isolate oneself
- hopelessness, helplessness, or worthlessness
- suddenly becoming calm or peaceful after a period of turmoil, especially if preceded by signs listed above (Robinson, 1989, p. 143)

Homicide

Homicide, death caused by one person ending another person's life, has the same characteristic of a sudden, unexpected, and helpless end to a relation-ship, but there are some differences. If the murderer is known, as is often the case, the family may have divided alliances, conflict, and anger. Guilt is evident in most cases of family violence that ends in homicide.

If the victim was killed in a robbery or the killer is unknown, rela-tives may also be in fear of their own lives. One young widow realized that her husband's killer, who was as yet unapprehended, had taken his address and house keys in the robbery. No one knew the reason for the murder. She was sure the killer would return to get her.

Healing for all of these people begins when they find out about the loss and can begin in the place the victim is pronounced dead, often an emergency room. Like the parents of the child who dies of SIDS, friends and family of suicide or homicide victims may need to spend time with the body, and to take some memento of the one who died. When it is not possible to see the body, as in the case of fire when the body is not recognizable, being in the same building or area where the body is may be helpful. They need information about legal issues, like autopsy requirements and when results will be known. There needs to be a place for them to meet with the police so that they can get information regarding property, suspects, and other issues. Clergy, family, and other people involved need to be called, so access to a phone is necessary. An institution that provides an environment in which these basic needs can be met is valued by the society it serves. Two women lost their husbands in a murder-robbery incident. The bodies were taken to two different hospitals for pronouncement of death. A few weeks later each new widow received a communication from the hospital to which her husband had been taken. The first widow opened the envelope and saw that she had received a bill for $75 for services rendered in the emergency room. The second widow opened the envelope and read a sensitively written letter expressing condolences for her loss, and offering referrals to grief counselors or hospital clergy. It is obvious that the second hospital, though also submitting a bill for services, is working to create a healing environment, and in this case, at almost no cost to the hospital. Nurses often take the lead in initiating this kind of effort.

Societal Issues

Social values in the United States are changing rapidly, and attitudes toward violence are a part of that change. Violence is an epidemic, and homicide is a major cause of death, especially among young people, disproportionately so among African American men. Increasing numbers of deaths of this kind move politicians and lawmakers to try measures like limiting the kinds of guns available to buy, increasing numbers of police on the streets, and providing more social programs to redirect young people to other kinds of life choices in handling anger and conflict.

Attitudes toward some kinds of suicide are changing, as well. Assisted suicide is becoming a political issue. The well-known Hemlock Society and Americans Against Human Suffering both promoted legislation (in California and Washington) that would make it legal to help people voluntarily commit suicide under very rigid guidelines. In some cases, the Washington initiative would make it legal to request and receive active, voluntary euthanasia (Quill, 1993). Oregon has passed such a referendum, allowing limited assisted suicide. The Oregon Circuit Court is becoming involved in interpreting the law. The legal issues are cloudy at this time. The National Hospice Organization and many local organizations have position statements on physician-assisted suicide.

Although society is in the process of defining values related to suicide and homicide, the survivors of victims of violence are confused and ambivalent. Support for the individuals is colored by an ever-changing view of the acceptability of violence. Shooting a person to death seems to be acceptable if the victim is engaged in a robbery on the shooter's premises or is threatening him in some way. Suicide is somewhat acceptable (and so families can be supported openly) if the victim was terminal, but rarely if the victim was depressed. The degree of guilt experienced by the family varies in part according to societal mores. Families and friends, the grief-stricken, are confused.

One way people deal with this kind of confusion is to take a stand and work on societal issues from the viewpoint of a victim or a family of a victim. Socially helpful ways of dealing with anger and guilt include joining (or forming) victims' rights groups, grassroots organizations for social change to help future generations avoid epidemics like the current violence. Examples of socially active groups that help in this way are Citizens Against Violence (CAVE), Families of Victims of Handguns, and People Against Rape (PAR). These and other groups provide a way to act out anger and change society in the direction a person believes it should go. Other people become politically active and work for specific legislation. Nurses, too, can use these groups to work for social change they feel is needed, and in doing so, work for healing of self and society.

THE DEATH OF A NURSE

When a nurse is terminally ill, other members of the health care team, and especially the nurses, are confronted by their own mortality in a very direct way. The dying nurse is a reminder of the fact that a caregiver is also human and is subject to the same rules of life and death as patients. For the nurse-caregiver who uses distance and separation from patients as a coping skill to protect from burnout and intense emotion, it may be impossible to care for a friend or other nurse. So, the nurse who is dying may be separated from the nurses who had formed a support system in both personal and professional life.

Professional caregivers may also want to render extraordinary care. Larry Dossey, M.D. (1993) wrote of being in bed with a back problem. Many of his professional friends came by to help him, but each had a different treatment or kind of care (like massage, imagery, and others) sure to help. In his case as in others, when a treatment is not chosen, the caregiver who offers it may feel rejected. A barrier may be created by loving people who cannot let the patient be in charge and accept the patient's choice of treatments. Caregivers have a hard time letting those they love make choices contrary to what they would have chosen.

Healing the dying nurse, like healing other dying individuals, focuses on relationships and comfort. Barriers to the dying nurse getting the same care needed by any dying patient include:

- fear of asking for help from others due to fear of being labeled a difficult patient
- recognition of difficulty of caregivers coping with care of a dying patient
- concerns about confidentiality of information
- belief that the nurses are too busy with people who can be helped to a greater degree (a way of continuing to care for others, even when dying)
- inconsistent or sporadic teaching, the health care team believing that the dying nurse has information she does not have
- insufficient rest, too many visitors

A dying nurse is a special person, needing the same care as other dying patients, but in a different way. Nurses believe that they know how the dying nurse feels. As with all perception, it must be validated by clear communication with the dying one, or it may be inaccurate. Honesty, the ability to allow the dying person to make choices contrary to the ones the caregiver would choose, and sensitivity to needs for visiting or rest, information or ventilation are critical components of caring for a person who is important in the community of nurses.

NEAR-DEATH EXPERIENCES

Dying people who discuss their near-death experiences (NDEs) with the nurses often become special to the nurses who care for them because their stories are so unique. Although the NDE may be either positive or negative to the person who experiences it, it usually helps the person to see meaning in life.

Some NDEs are not particularly dramatic. One police officer who was shot and being treated in a trauma center remembers floating above her body, watching the team cut off her clothes, and realizing how sick she was. But she immediately found herself back in her body, and in her fight to get well forgot the NDE entirely until a nurse asked her if she had experienced anything strange or unusual during her illness. Her NDE stimulated her to wonder what happened, to examine the seriousness of her illness, and to consider what happens after death. It did not change her life in any appreciable way, but it started her investigation into the meaning of her own life.

A dock worker who was in a near-fatal accident was also asked about unusual experiences, and broke down and began to cry. He told of going through a dark tunnel, reaching a beautiful new land. In that bright and peaceful place, he saw and talked with white-robed figures and his dead mother. After several more experiences there, he returned to his pain-filled body and hoped to die so he could reenter the land. Once he was out of the intensive care unit, he told his wife of his experience, but he told no health care workers until the nurse gave him the opportunity. This man had a very emotional experience and was already planning how to change his life. His wife was supportive of the changes, which included church membership and a new interest in community activities.

Both of these patients believed they had come close to death and survived. Both verbalized that they no longer feared death, though the process of pain and separation from loved ones was still upsetting. Both of them needed to talk with someone who believed their unique experiences and could simply listen, without ascribing meaning beyond the incident. That is, the nurse neither glorified the incident, nor minimized it. The experience a person has when he comes close to death is not death itself. Therefore, one cannot support nor deny the concept of life after death as it was described by a person who has experienced an NDE. Life after death is a matter of faith, not science. The NDE suggests that there may be peace and much more than we understand at the moment of death, and it can be a comfort to families to know that a loved one has experienced such an event. Each experience is unique and has unique meaning to the person who experiences it.

Care of the person who has experienced an NDE includes:

- listening without judgment
- helping the person to share the story with family
- referral to clergy or spiritual guide if requested
- counseling, if the person is planning to change direction in life and that direction is contrary to the family's values
- introducing the person to others who have had the experience, if others are available, to form a small support group

Sometimes when caring for a person who is dying, the nurse hears the person relate the experience of becoming peaceful and no longer fearing death because of an NDE. If the family is not present when this occurs, the nurse has the opportunity to share the experience with them, and it often gives much comfort to them, to know that the person died in peace. Other visions the dying person may relate, like the presence of a dead family member, may be shared with family for whatever meaning they have to them.

SUMMARY

Every life is unique, every person special. This chapter is about people who are special because they are members of a particular group of people who require special care when they are dying. We care differently for people who are our family or friends, who are stigmatized or have diseases we fear, who are vulnerable, as children are, or who have special stories that help us to search for our own meaning in life. We care differently for their families and loved ones, because they have different needs.

Every nurse must take the time to know herself, to know if her own coping depends upon separating herself from dying friends or avoiding difficult situations. Every nurse needs to know if fear of AIDS or other disease interferes with the care of those who have the disease. Every nurse needs to be able to listen to and support the patient with unique deathbed experiences.

REFERENCES

Akner, L. (1993). *How to survive the loss of a parent.* New York: William Morrow and Co.

Anonymous (1998). *Hospice care: A physicians guide.* Raleigh, NC: National Hospice Organization.

Benoliel, J. Q. (1991). Multiple meanings of death for older adults. In E. M. Baines (Ed.) *Perspectives on gerontological nursing.* Newbury Park, CA: Sage Publications.

Bouman, C. C. (1994). Nursing management of adults with immune disorders. In P. Beare & J. Myers (Eds.), *Principles and practice of adult health nursing* (2nd ed.). St. Louis, MO: C. V. Mosby Year-Book, Inc.

Buckingham, R. (1990). *Care of the dying child.* New York: Continuum.

Corr, C. A., Fuller, H., Barnickol, C. A., & Corr, D. M. (1991). *Sudden infant death syndrome: Who can help and how.* New York: Springer Publishing Co.

Dolce, L. (1992). *Suicide.* New York: Chelsea House Publishers.

Dossey, L. (1993). *Healing words.* San Francisco: HarperCollins.

El-Sadr, W., Oleske, J. M., & Agins, B. D., (1994). *Evaluation and management of early HIV infection. Clinical practice guideline no. 7* (AHCPR Publication No. 94-0572). Rockville, MD: Agency for Health Care Policy and Research, Public Health Service, U.S. Department of Health and Human Services.

Lester, D. (1993). *The enigma of adolescent suicide.* Philadelphia: The Charles Press.

Moffat, B. C. (1986). *When someone you love has AIDS.* New York: NAL Penguin.

Quill, T. (1993). *Death and dignity: Making choices and taking charge.* New York: W. W. Norton & Co.

Robinson, R. (1989). *Survivors of suicide.* Santa Monica, CA: IBS Press.

White, R., & Cunningham, A. M. (1991). *Ryan White: My own story.* New York: Dial Books.

CHAPTER 11

Those Who Care for the Dying

CARING FOR DYING PEOPLE

Death overload is a term that indicates that a caregiver has experienced the death of too many patients in a short period or too much personal investment in patients for too long a time (Vachon, 1993). For nurses who started one palliative care unit, their distress scores were equal to those of newly widowed women and higher than those of women with newly diagnosed breast cancer who were undergoing radiation therapy. Yet in other studies, nurses who cared for people with life-threatening illnesses, including hospice nurses, had less distress and more coping skills than nurses in other fields. Some nurses clearly have the ability to grow into the role of caring for dying people in a way that supports their own growth and expert practice, and to change the environment so that it can support other caregivers to do the same. It is important for all professional caregivers who care for the dying to clearly understand the emotional risks to themselves and plan to use the experience to nurture their spirit and develop the ability to be present in each moment, savoring life in its fullest, and finding meaning in being there for the dying patient.

One Model of Occupational Stress

Vachon (1987) developed a model of occupational stress based on Antonovsky's definition of stress. Stress is "a demand made by the internal or external environment of the organism that upsets its homeostasis, restoration of which depends upon a non-automatic and not readily available energy-expending action" (Antonovsky, 1979, p. 162). In this model, stress is different from routine stimuli, and it is different for different people. Routine stimuli may become stressful if the balance of the environment is upset. One death on a nursing unit where death is a likely prognosis may be a routine stimulus. Several deaths in a day or a week may upset the environment of the unit, cause disruption in the ability of those present to hope, to plan for care, and to grieve sufficiently for each dying person.

According to Antonovsky, in order to reestablish the routine in this scenario, the nurses must take some action. For the nurses to go on as if nothing had happened means that the normal pattern of caregiving, the camaraderie, the gestalt of the unit will be adversely affected, morale will suffer, and death overload or burnout will occur among the staff. Vachon's model helps identify the areas of action that can help.

Simply stated, the occupational stress model explains that job stress is the consequence of the interaction of personal characteristics with the environment over time. To affect the consequences of job stress, including burnout or overload, one must act on either personal characteristics or the environment or both. Personal characteristics that influence the perception of an individual nurse, leading to an evaluation of the event as stressful include:

- age—younger nurses have developed fewer coping skills and see events as more stressful

- personality, including motivation for caring for the dying, personal value system, coping style, and skills

- previous and current stressful life events, especially experience caring for dying people, both as a nurse and as a family member or friend

- social support from other professional colleagues, as well as from friends and family outside the profession

There are many motivations for caring for the dying or otherwise vulnerable people. Each of these motivating characteristics can be a source of strength or a source of stress. Motivation for caring for the dying may come from a deep set of values demanding action on behalf of suffering people, perhaps as a call of faith, or a desire to improve the world. But if a nurse (or other health care provider) is motivated to care for the dying because of the unresolved death of a loved one, the nurse is particularly at risk. Other unresolved deaths are likely to lead to distress and burnout. A positive outcome would be that the stress itself becomes a motivating factor to resolve the family losses.

Hardiness is a personality characteristic that is helpful to patients and nurses alike. A hardy person has a sense of commitment, a sense of meaningfulness, physical or psychological endurance, the power to influence events, boldness, and a feeling of challenge. Conversely, the person who is not hardy is alienated, powerless, threatened, and has little sense of goal directedness. Hardy nurses and hardy patients can work together by sharing control and decision making in planning care. These characteristics create a powerful impetus for individuals to create an environment or an atmosphere of healing.

A nurse's support system also influences the perception of burnout or stress following the death of one or more patients. If a nurse's support comes mainly from a social group, there may be a lack of understanding of the depth of his feelings about the events at work. In addition, his social group may not want to hear about sad or difficult times, may not want to provide the needed listening ear or be available to cry with the nurse who is sad. If the grief is a regular occurrence, friends get tired of hearing about it, though they are often willing to provide needed distraction. A group of professional people with whom the nurse can share the losses may be more helpful. They are more likely to understand, to have experiences that can be usefully shared, and to have coping skills that are helpful to the nurse who has lost a patient. They know when to recommend a different course of action like taking time off or creating a bereavement group.

Other personal characteristics that leave the individual caregiver vulnerable to the particular stressors of caring for dying people include family variables. Birth order (the eldest child), gender (female in most cultures), and a family history of substance or other abuse predispose some people to continue their role of caregiver. An eldest, female, adult child in a dysfunctional family is often attracted to a caregiving role, and any of the health care professions, like nursing, social work, physical therapy, and medicine provide that opportunity. Anyone who comes from a dysfunctional family may continue the dysfunctional behaviors of the family in professional life when stress is severe.

Environmental characteristics that predispose caregivers working in that environment to experience tension and poor coping skills related to stress include:

- poor communication patterns with other caregivers in the area, and with patients and their families
- role overload, role strain, and role ambiguity
- inadequate resources and staffing (adapted from Vachon, 1993)

Poor communication patterns not only predispose the nurse and others to the consequences of occupational stress, but have been documented to be harmful to patients (Baggs, Ryan, Phelps, Richeson, & Johnson, 1993). For nurses, the inability to discuss patients adequately with physicians often means that they feel unable to get appropriate care for the patient, such as medication orders or other treatment. The physician may feel frustrated at not having the knowledge about the patient on which to base decisions, such as whether new medications are necessary. The other staff, therapists, personal care aids, and consultants all try to function without needed information. Professional rivalry develops. Team members form coalitions and factions begin to form, with conflict soon following.

Communication problems with patient and family are stressful because the patient may not be able to express need, so the team cannot meet that need. The family may blame the staff and physician for the patient's failing health. Ultimately, caring for this individual is not satisfying because it becomes a source of constant conflict. A lack of trust between all parties develops.

Role strain, overload, and ambiguity are all stressors with which nurses in many settings are familiar. Role strain occurs when one has difficulty performing all the required aspects of one's role. This may be related to lack of information, as when there are communication problems and all the relevant information is not available. Lack of knowledge about what to do or how to do it (as when pain control is inadequate, and one does not know what to do) may be a factor. Or lack of resources to complete the tasks or make the best choices for the care of an individual may be the cause of a nurse not performing all the aspects of the role satisfactorily.

Role overload occurs when one feels that there is just too much to do. Nurses tend to try to finish, no matter what the job, often staying late, charting after hours, and becoming frustrated and tired. This is particularly identified as stressful if it is required by others or not taken on willingly by the health care worker. For example, most nurses do not mind staying late because a patient needs to talk about a problem or there is a need to contact a doctor about a new order. But if the case load as assigned is consistently greater than safe staffing ratios permit, it is role overload, and leads to people feeling stressed.

Role ambiguity and role conflict are the result of not knowing what the role really involves, and what another person's role includes. This problem reflects the fact that the role expectations are not clearly defined in the system. Advanced nurse practitioners are prone to this kind of problem. A pain management specialist may be called for medication titration, education of staff in pain assessment, management of epidural medication systems, writing policies, presenting information to physicians, massage, and imagery. To do all of these things well is very difficult, and may lead to role overload, but without knowing what the expectations of the role are, it is hard to choose which of those tasks are most urgent, which are the priorities. Role conflict is experienced when the individual's many roles in life conflict, as when one's professional life conflicts with personal goals. An example occurs when one is asked to be on call during a time when the family has been promised an outing.

The fear of inadequate resources is related to the current health care financing crisis, and it is a reality in some health care settings. There is always a dynamic tension between the provision of high-quality care, which requires resources, and the need to restrain costs in health care, which have been rising much faster than inflation for many years. Limited dollars do not automatically mean that care will be substandard. Unfortunately, when resources are limited, staff is often limited, and psychosocial care is sacrificed. For the dying patient, that is a critical aspect of care, and nurses feel care is substandard if it is not available. Professional health care providers in any discipline who cannot provide the kind of care they believe is important, especially to people with terminal illness, are going to experience the consequences of job-related stress.

Consequences of Stress for Providers of Care

Stress-related problems, like the causes of the stress, are related to the system, the individual, or both. Coping mechanisms used to handle stress-related problems are those things one does to make the system supportive to staff and those things one does to care for self.

One young nurse tearfully turned in her resignation to her supervisor after the death of the third patient that week. She told the supervisor that she could not cope with death, that she could not sleep, eat, or stop thinking about one of the patients. This nurse was sure she could have done more for all of them, especially one who died unexpectedly. She felt "so sorry for the three-year-old who lost his mother" that she bought him a stuffed rabbit, then could not give it to him. Her spiritual distress was becoming all-consuming.

This nurse exemplified many consequences of stress. Caregivers of dying people reexamine their own belief systems, sometimes suffering an existential crisis of faith. They grieve each loss, and if the losses come too quickly, they do not complete their grieving before the next death. Other common feelings include:

- guilt
- anger
- irritability
- frustration
- helplessness
- inadequacy
- sleeplessness
- depression

These feelings may lead to problems with interactions with patients, family, and other staff. To cope with increasing pressure, this nurse admitted that she had avoided contact with new patients, reasoning that the patients she knew needed her more. Intellectualizing her actions in this way reinforced her feelings of inadequacy because she knew her assessments were not complete, and she did not work toward establishing the trust that newly diagnosed, terminally ill patients needed. She avoided meaningful contact with individual patients by making rounds with other staff or while the patients were asleep. Her judgment suffered, omitting referrals that were obviously needed, making others that were not. All of this reinforced her sense of guilt, and she became evasive with her coworkers, flaring in anger when asked to stay late. Her fiance resented her constant funereal conversation, wanting to know when she would begin to laugh again. Finally, she agreed with him that resignation was the way out of the dilemma. Results of the feelings experienced by nurses who are not coping well with the deaths of patients may include clinical problems like:

- avoiding the patient
- poor clinical judgment
- unrealistic expectations
- staff absences
- outbursts of anger
- lack of anticipatory planning
- staff conflict
- scapegoating
- interdisciplinary power struggles
- staff fatigue
- ambivalence toward patients

Two things need to happen for the young nurse to grow in her ability to care for the dying and to find satisfaction, even joy, in doing so. The first is that she learns to care for herself. The second is that the environment, including the institution or organization she is associated with and people she works with, becomes energetic, supportive, and healing.

CHANGING THE ENVIRONMENT

Leadership skills are required to change the environment. Policy and politics are not bad words, and the ability to use them is necessary for change to happen. Politics is defined here as: to gain and use enough power to get done what needs to be done. This may mean forming coalitions with other groups of caregivers to make policies that work. For example, one group of nurses was having difficulty getting the anesthesia team to respond quickly when called for pain management. Instead of complaining to each other and becoming frustrated by the situation, they carefully documented the time lag between calls to the service and response for a month. They presented their information to their supervisor (called an outcomes manager in that system) who was responsible for quality assurance. That manager gave the information to three attending physicians who regularly admitted patients to that special care unit. At the same time, the nurses on the unit had developed reasonable goals for response time and a policy that set out a plan by which nurses could get help when needed for patient pain management, who was responsible, and what to do if the team did not respond. A team meeting between the anesthesia team, attending physicians, a patient advocate (ombudsman), and nursing representation quickly adopted the policy change. The anesthesia team began responding within defined time limits, and when one of them did not, the policy as adopted was used and the anesthesia department intervened to provide the help the nurses needed to provide care. This is an example of the appropriate use of politics—forming coalitions between members of various groups to change policy to meet defined goals.

Another leadership skill is the ability to recognize when staff ideas have merit and should be supported, even if resources are scarce. Staff may recognize when support groups of various kinds are needed, and when they have become routine and outlived their usefulness. In either case, the ability to begin programs like support groups and discontinue them when they have served their purpose should be a clinical decision, and policy should not make those decisions difficult to carry out. Nurse managers can support initiative and change, helping staff who have ideas with merit to implement them.

Team building is another skill nurse managers use to create an environment of healing. Nurses who care for the dying sometimes need an extra day off, help in caring for a difficult patient, or other considerations. Some nurses should not be assigned to a certain kind of patient based on feelings related to family history. For example, a nurse may be unable to care for a burn patient if a family member was in a fire and there are unresolved feelings about that incident. Consideration for assignment change and an occasional mental health day are ways of recognizing unique needs of staff members.

Nurse colleagues need to know and accept the fact that each of them will need that consideration and be willing to provide it for others. That willingness to stand in for colleagues only comes if the members of the staff who work together trust each other to use requests for help only when needed. Most staff members will become resentful of another member of the staff who:

- asks for help with every difficult patient

- takes time off from work for family convenience

- does not make an effort to resolve the problems that put up barriers to caring for some patients

- requests special consideration more often than seems indicated

A needy staff person will become isolated and possibly disruptive to the rest of the staff, calling in sick more often and in other ways attempting to meet needs for self-care that interrupt the flow of the team effort to create a special environment.

Team building requires that all members of the team agree on a few basic principles. The first is to decide who the members of the team are. The nursing team (whether a home care group, a hospice group, a hospital group, or other) is a team nested within a larger organization, and the whole health care team should have an identity. The whole team should have a sense of purpose, of goals that are shared, and how those goals will be met. A mutual respect for other team members and their abilities is a prerequisite to a trusting relationship and the ability to leave a task in another person's hands. Members of different professions sometimes have overlapping competencies. That is, a nurse, a clergyperson, and a social worker may all have skill in counseling a patient regarding an identified spiritual need. But if they all try to counsel one patient, that person may be confused or refuse the ministrations of one or two members of the team, leading to hurt feelings. It is better for the team members to recognize the abilities of each other, have a plan for deciding who does what (including the patient's choice), and trust that the person doing the work can do it well. If the care provider does not request help with the task, the other care providers should not attempt to intervene (or rescue the team member) even if they think they could do it better. Although there are times when a knowledgeable person can suggest alternate ways of approaching a problem, criticizing the person entrusted with the care of the patient often creates distrust and conflict. Offering to help is acceptable if the environment as a whole is supportive to the workers, and the offer is not likely to be viewed as interference or distrust. The team may agree that there are many right ways to do something.

Fostering an atmosphere of mutual support makes it possible for all the staff to put into words their feelings about the care they give and the people for whom they care. Regular team meetings allow problem solving for patient care issues, as well as the identification of problems staff members may be developing in relation to that care. The well-functioning team can point out to the stressed nurse what seems to be happening so that the nurse can assess the situation and move to change it. Or the team may offer to take on some responsibility for care if overload is a contributing factor. The group may help each other understand why a particular patient makes them angry or makes them feel guilty. Sometimes an outside support person, like a visiting psychologist or a psychiatric consultation liaison nurse, may help the group dynamics, so the team does not become negative.

A mutually supportive environment is one perceived by patients and staff as a healing environment. Such an environment is built on trust, recognition of the skills and abilities of colleagues, a leadership that can accomplish appropriate change and attract needed resources, and the establishment of a kind of unique gestalt, or special feeling about the place and its people. That special feeling is easy to recognize, hard to define. People in such environments greet each other (and strangers) warmly, often with smiles. Though incredibly busy, they are not short tempered or sour in demeanor. There is a frequent use of humor, but not dark humor that risks offending people. People are able to laugh at their situations, sometimes even at the physical changes in themselves. Family and visitors soon pick up the feeling. There are instances of a whole group of people (not usually staff) arriving at the room of a person who has lost all hair due to treatment with their heads shaved in a show of support. Staff members can laugh with the group, encourage the camaraderie, have the group visit other bald patients, and join in the fun.

These environments are also creative. No two are alike. The main feelings are caring, serenity, and love. There is an intention to help other people, a desire to make a difference. There is a clear sense of purpose. That is expressed in spontaneous conversations—begun with a statement like, "How shall we help Mrs. K?" Patients feel free to ask for the help they need. The healing environment for the nurse includes policies that support the ability to take a day off when needed, or to arrange for a group meeting for the purposes of sharing care problems and frustrations. The ability to get a facilitator for the group can be helpful.

The physical environment is both stimulating and serene, accomplished by having things like plants, colorful pictures, music of different types at different times, balloons when celebrating, and quiet when peace is needed. Personal items belonging to both staff and patients may be present. For staff, the items may be pictures on walls, helpful books, photographs of previous patients, awards, or other remembrances. For patients, photographs and personal items with special meaning are there. People get together in small groups. Some people spontaneously hug others, and those who do not like to hug shake hands or receive a pat on the back as a more acceptable way to make physical contact. In some settings, a separate room is available for private conversations, meditation, and prayer, a private telephone, reading materials, special rituals, or crying.

Healing environments can be found in places like the waiting room of an intensive care unit, the outpatient department of a large urban hospital, nursing centers for primary care, hospice units or organizations, or specialty care settings, like transplant units or oncology centers. When they exist, both patients and nurses are able to experience healing.

The health care system continues to be constrained by financial pressures because of policies by health maintenance organizations, cuts in Medicare/Medicaid, and the like. Large health care systems are closing because of financial exigencies. People caring for the dying may believe that resources to implement self-care strategies are politically and financially untenable. However, studies of the administration of services show that employees who perceive they have access to empowerment structures, like support, resources, information, and opportunity, have less job tension and increased work effectiveness. Employees are more productive and meet both patient and organizational goals (Laschinger, Wong, McMahon, & Kaufmann, 1999). Gage (1998) calls for "total stakeholder satisfaction." Synergistic health care teams function for the patient, the members, and the organization. Changing the environment to one of healing and nurturing is cost effective.

CARING FOR SELF

Wise, mature, expert nurses root their care for others in healthy life patterns for themselves. They have knowledge of their strengths and self-confidence in their abilities. They have confronted their own mortality, and have developed a philosophy of life that is compatible with the choice they have made to work with dying people. The death of a patient is not viewed as a failure. They see each moment in life as an opportunity to make choices of some kind, for good.

Keegan (1994) suggests that the most important category of attributes of healers, including nurses, is attitude because it is from attitude that people act. That attitude is grounded in a sense of meaning and purpose in life, a sense of becoming empowered by service to others, a sense of one's place in the natural world, and an ability to use one's life experiences (even the sad ones) in the care of others. Nurses who do this are recognized by their joy, caring spirit, clear sense of purpose, and intent to use hands, heart, and spirit. They are hands-on, empathetic, genuine, centered, and connected people.

Motivation

The question "Why care for people who are dying?" is important. For any provider of care to become a healer of the dying, identifying motivation is important. Occasionally a nurse who has been caring for the terminally ill for some time has a sudden realization that caring for these people is an attempt to answer questions for himself about difficult instances in life. The nurse must identify the fact that unresolved issues in life can be barriers to care and to happiness and joy in the work. When the nurse realizes that unresolved problems exist, it is important to confront those issues in a useful way by requesting the help of a professional counselor, a competent spiritual guide, or a knowledgeable colleague who has the expertise to help.

A second nurse may be professionally challenged by the many ways available to help dying people both in physical care for comfort and for care beyond the physical that involves search for meaning and peace. This nurse may be passing through the palliative care model, later using skills learned from the lessons the dying have to teach with other patients who may not be dying. This nurse is intellectually stimulated by palliative care.

Another nurse in the same area revels in the growth of each patient as that person comes to terms with the nature of mortality and the beauty of life in many forms. This nurse is a nurturer, a person who is likely to use a creative approach to help people achieve their own goals. This nurse may also care for the dying as a manifestation of service to humankind, a spiritual calling to be fulfilled, intrigued and compelled by each individual's search for meaning in life.

Yet another nurse may find joy in the physical care of very ill people, using a variety of techniques found to be effective in the care of dying people, like massage, yoga, breathing exercises, Therapeutic Touch, and others. This nurse probably cares for herself in a similar way, taking classes in aerobic exercises or T'ai Chi, maintaining an active life-style.

The motivations for each of these nurses are not mutually exclusive. The nurse-healer strives for balance, growing in all of life by understanding how his feelings influence his actions with patients. This nurse learns new and useful skills of communication. He learns systems of exercises and comfort measures. He actively maintains his physical health to help sustain energy and hardiness. This nurse also works to develop a rich spiritual life, maintaining connections with his inner self and the larger universe. A healer may focus on one area for a while, then move to a different level of growth as a result of an experience with a dying patient.

Coping Techniques

Coping skills include anything one can use to alter the relationship between the person and the environment to change the negative results of psychophysiologic consequences of stress. Ted is an example of using forgiveness as a means of coping with a set of feelings that had been negative in his life for years.

Ted

Ted was an RN with four years of experience on a general medical hospital unit. Patients on the unit had a variety of serious diagnoses, and many of them died. One patient reminded Ted of an aunt who had died when he was five years old. That was also the age when he began school. The death of his aunt became linked with the abandonment he felt when his parents left him at the school door. Venting his feelings about the patient to a supervisor, Ted suddenly realized that the onset of his poor job performance (which he had labeled as burnout) was related to his feelings about this past experience. He decided to talk over how he felt with his parents, and to tell himself he forgave them for the perceived abandonment. This simple insight and related action helped Ted to consider forgiveness as an important conscious way to deal with hidden grudges and negative feelings about others. This gave him a new way of relating to other staff, and brought him new joy in his work. He worked on letting go of bad feelings about others by simply forgiving them, without regard to assigning blame. Forgiveness for Ted became a coping mechanism.

There are a number of techniques that help professionals who are caring for dying patients stay healthy. Maintaining their balance between a philosophy that helps to give meaning to what they are doing and growing in ability to confront personal challenge is one goal. Continuing the kind of connection with others that leads to service is another.

Maintaining health is the first important coping technique nurses use to combat the special stressors of caring for the dying. There are many physical strategies used to enhance the health of both nurses and patients who feel stressed. Obviously, good nutrition and weight control, regular exercise, adequate sleep, and sufficient resources to maintain these things are important.

Vigorous exercise is helpful because it contributes to good weight control and helps develop strength and endurance. Exercise initiates biochemical changes that support one's ability to feel tranquil and peaceful after the exercise, and provides a time to be away from the source of the stressor. A regular schedule of well-chosen exercises that are both physically challenging and pleasurable is most likely to be continued over time.

Other kinds of physical activities that are useful coping strategies include massage, diaphragmatic breathing, and distraction. Each of these techniques must fit into a program of general time management, valuing time for self as well as competent, planned patient-care time management. Massage is a technique used for many years by nurses for patients. But at least one nursing department invested in a massage chair for staff! Nurses knowledgeable in massage techniques help each other with periodic 15-minute neck and shoulder massages. Release of muscle tension in shoulders and back breaks the feeling of stress, refreshes, and relaxes. Time is scheduled, allowing nurses to anticipate a period of focus on themselves. The brief time of focus on the caregiver in a practical, caring way reinforces a caring environment and gives the nurses a respite in an otherwise busy day of focus on others.

Diaphragmatic breathing is a useful technique to learn for relaxing and to begin the centering process. Consciously realizing the path each inhalation takes through the respiratory passages, and allowing each breath to move to the bottom of the respiratory tree by moving the diaphragm downward and outward moves the whole person toward feeling more relaxed. As the slow, long exhalation occurs, a person feels shoulders moving downward and tension slowly leaving the body. To help with stress at work, a nurse should practice diaphragmatic breathing at home, in either a supine or sitting position. Putting one's hand on the abdomen is an easy way to know if the abdomen is involved in the breath, or if shallow, tense breaths are a pattern. Once a pattern of abdominal breathing is the norm, the nurse can think words like, "I can feel this way whenever I take a deep breath and cross my fingers." Connecting the relaxed feeling to the physical act of crossing fingers (or any other physical cue) helps the body to remember how it feels to relax. A nurse who regularly practices this technique has the ability to break the cycle of stress and muscle tension identified even at the bedside of a dying patient in just a few seconds. The pattern is:

- recognize the feeling of tension
- take an abdominal breath
- use a physical cue that has been practiced
- allow shoulders to sag and relaxation to be experienced during the exhalation

This technique, or pattern, is useful by itself to help relax for a few minutes or to lead to more profound states of relaxation. For the nurse who is attempting to help the patient by using Healing Touch or some other energy work, breathing from the diaphragm helps to become focused. It helps a nurse to move to a place of peace within, an awareness of the space created between patient and nurse that is healing to both people in this unique relationship. Diaphragmatic breathing may also be a way of centering, or an adjunctive technique to other forms of relaxation, including:

- progressive muscle relaxation (PMR)
- autogenic relaxation
- sentic cycles
- relaxation imagery
- meditation in many forms

Nurses who practice diaphragmatic breathing for a time often go on to learn other relaxation techniques that become a consistent resource for dealing with stress and tension. Practice sessions should occur at least three times a day, for five to ten minutes a session. Within a week or two, the skill will be learned. With continued practice, the ability to relax will deepen. Relaxation techniques are defined in Table 11-1.

Distraction is another coping technique, which is necessary to break a pattern of tension, to get away from an intense situation if only for a few seconds. Humor, a deep breath, a massage break, someone's story about a family member or a book recently read, or a lunch break can serve as a useful distraction, allowing the nurse to come back to the situation with a fresh viewpoint and perhaps more energy. A heavy work

---

TABLE 11-1 **Relaxation Techniques**

Progressive muscle relaxation

Alternately tensing and relaxing skeletal muscles, starting with the feet and going through each major muscle group. Concentration is on feeling the difference between a tense and a relaxed muscle group. The tension phase is omitted when one is comfortable in knowing what relaxation feels like.

Autogenic relaxation

Mentally repeating phrases scripted to reflect the sensations of a relaxed body, such as "Each muscle is relaxed and limp."

Sentic cycles

Mentally rehearsing a series of intense emotions, alternating opposite emotions, such as peace with anger.

Imagery

Using an internal process, the imager explores various senses, such as vision, auditory, kinesthetic, and other senses.

Meditation

An inner process of listening to that which is inside oneself and which connects with the universe. Depending upon the type of practice, meditation can be a relaxation technique, an altered state of consciousness, a hypometabolic state, or a spiritual practice, such as contemplative prayer or a type of yoga.

schedule should not be used as an excuse to avoid a lunch break. Although it may be necessary to make a meal a short one, it is most often true that a nurse who has been away from an intense situation for a few minutes is able to return feeling more able to help. Family members, too, need to be encouraged to take a break, or a deep breath, or tell a story now and then to decrease the tension in the environment.

If a long, intense relationship comes to an end through the death of a favorite patient or someone for whom it has been a significant challenge to care, the distraction may need to be longer, perhaps a day off or a vacation to rest and refresh one's spirit. Planning to use that time as fun, scheduling things that are not reminders of a patient or death and dying may be important, and may be alternated with the need to grieve, attend services or final rituals, and remember significant people, including patients, in one's life.

DEVELOPING THE SPIRITUAL SELF

Knowing that one's life has meaning and confronting one's mortality are the key elements in developing the ability to care for people who are dying. A nurse who has not identified a reason for being does not have direction in life and a framework for action. It is easy to get distracted from any sense of purpose, pulled from a moment of joy into someone's problems, another's loss, a third person's fears. *Healing the dying* means healing oneself by forming connections with the Universe and all that it is. It means a path one can count on, a way one travels with confidence, accompanied by others for parts of the journey.

A search for meaning need not be a lonely search, a sad or intellectual search. In fact, learning to listen is the most important requirement. The use of quiet, peaceful environments like gardens or meditation rooms is useful for quieting the chatter of the mind, hearing the whisper of nature, of the inner self, and connecting to one's own spirituality.

A structure or discipline of some kind is useful, for it provides landmarks by which to gauge progress. For example, people who grow up regularly attending religious services have gone through consistent rites of passage, moving to new religious education classes each year, having

One Tired Nurse

Samantha was tired, frustrated, and felt like being alone. She decided her spirit was tired and needed renewal. Life seemed hard. She planned a weekend retreat at a monastery that offered guest cottages and quiet gardens in which to walk. During the weekend, the Catholic monks invited this Protestant woman (the only woman on the grounds) to their regular services. Samantha accepted, thinking the music would assist her search for peace. She was surprised when they offered her a seat in the choir (the section of pews where the monks sit). When the monks went to the altar for communion services, she stayed in her seat, knowing that the rite was reserved for those of the Catholic faith. One of the monks came to her and said, "Why don't you come with us, just for a hug." Suddenly, her spirit soared. Seeking a weekend of solitude and peace, she found a community with a spirit that resonated with hers. They were united in a mutual caring, the beauty of the place, the music, and God. Samantha does not need to return to the monastery to feel the joy and to know there is a bridge between the present and the unseen.

ceremonies indicating movement toward adulthood (like confirmation of faith, public expression of conversion, bar mitzvah), and joining groups of like-minded people on the search. When the inner development does not keep pace with the group's development, a person is likely to drop out, sometimes returning later. Inner development is supported by studies, the culture or religious group, and group and individual reflection on faith.

For some people, organized religion is not the road to a sense of connection with meaningfulness and purpose. Sometimes they attain an abiding spiritual focus by connections with nature. A walk along the oceanfront, a long hike in the mountains, or a meditative session next to a waterfall all provide a sense of oneness with nature and a knowledge of belonging to the community of humankind and the Universe. One's purpose is in being.

Whether one seeks a spiritual awakening within a group or as an individual, the path is an inner process. Whether one achieves a transforming moment, a peak experience always to be remembered, or proceeds through the process a little at a time, learning through each contact with each person, there is a growing sense of unity and purpose in being. One belongs here. One has a mission, a service. One is committed to a path of action.

There are many ways one can choose to develop a deeper spirituality or an ability to listen to the inner self. Other than formal association with a spiritual group, they include:

- learning to meditate or pray
- creating an environment that supports peace—using nature, music, or sounds like waterfalls or ocean waves, art or furniture, like a kneeling bench, or cushions to sit on
- reading literature that teaches how to develop a spiritual path, and biographies of those known for their spiritual natures
- setting a regular time to practice whichever form of discipline one chooses
- keeping a spiritual journal, or diary
- sharing one's journey with other spiritually mature people
- guiding other people in spiritual journeys
- enjoying life

SUMMARY

All people who care for terminally ill patients are at risk for developing a special kind of distress related to the many losses and an incomplete understanding of the role. They also have the potential for developing a life of service leading to great joy, a feeling of professional and personal competence, and an ability to live their own lives to the fullest. It is a matter of choice.

The person who chooses to grow through the experience of caring for others actively maintains a balance between all areas of good health: exercise, nutrition, sleep, social support, deepening friendships, commitment, and a clear sense of a spiritual journey, a connection with all of life through all generations. An understanding of one's meaning in life leads to the ability to enjoy it. Those who enjoy it can share it.

REFERENCES

Antonovsky, A. (1979). *Health, stress and coping*. San Francisco: Jossey-Bass.

Baggs, J. D., Ryan, S. A., Phelps, C. E., Richeson, F., & Johnson, J. E. (1993). Collaboration in critical care. *Heart & Lung, 21*(1), 18–24.

Gage, M. (1998). From independence to interdependence. *Journal of Nursing Administration, 28*(4), 17–26.

Keegan, L. (1994). *The nurse as healer*. New York: Delmar Publishers.

Laschinger, H. K., Wong, C., McMahon, L., & Kaufmann, C. (1999). Leader behavior impact on staff nurse empowerment, job tension and work effectiveness. *Journal of Nursing Administration, 29*(5), 28–39.

Vachon, M. L. (1987). *Occupational stress in the care of the critically ill, the dying and the bereaved*. New York: Hemisphere.

Vachon, M. L. (1993). Emotional problems in palliative medicine: patient, family and professional. In D. Doyle, G. Hanks, & N. MacDonald (Eds.), *Oxford textbook of palliative medicine* (pp. 577–605). Oxford: Oxford University Press.

Epilogue

Ms. F. left the V.A. Hospital to go to school. Two weeks after she left, she was eating breakfast and reading the paper. Mr. Bower popped into her memory, and she wondered how he was doing. She remembered how he waited for her each evening, so often with a small issue, no really transcendent moments, nothing dramatic or memorable. Yet through the eight-month period that she had known him, he had changed. They had developed a special relationship that was satisfying and healing for each of them at different times. She remembered how he had helped when Luke died, giving up his room, and later telling her that she did well, helping her self-confidence and her sense of competency in her work.

He continued to question, to learn, to help his comrades, to become more settled and satisfied with life. He knew he would die, fought it for a time, and became progressively more peaceful. He had learned that he did not want to give up and would continue to do what he could to live well. He made peace with his God and with his family. He also made many plans. He made a will and left his medals to his newly found grandson. He shared this news with the men on his unit, and they rejoiced with him. He knew he had made a difference in life, that his life had meaning because of his wartime contributions. He had learned to be satisfied with his life, glad he had lived it.

Then Ms. F. read the small headline. It said, "P. Bower, war hero, dies of cancer." The notice went on to say he had died the night before. It listed his daughter and her family as next of kin. And there was a paragraph about his silver star and his heroism in saving lives of others.

Ms. F. had not realized the extent of his heroism. After a few moments of grief and sadness, she smiled. His temporal life was closed, but he had taught her how it was to die. She felt he left more of a legacy than he realized as her teacher, and she was glad. It had been a healing relationship.

Haight's Life Review and Experiencing Form

CHILDHOOD

1. What is the very first thing you can remember in your life? Go as far back as you can.

2. What other things can you remember about when you were very young?

3. What was life like for you as a child?

4. What were your parents like? What were their weaknesses, strengths?

5. Did you have any brothers or sisters? Tell me what each was like.

6. Did someone close to you die when you were growing up?

7. Did someone important to you go away?

8. Do you ever remember being very sick?

9. Do you remember having an accident?

10. Do you remember being in a very dangerous situation?

11. Was there anything that was important to you that was lost or destroyed?

12. Was church a large part of your life?

13. Did you enjoy being a boy/girl?

ADOLESCENCE

1. When you think about yourself and your life as a teenager, what is the first thing you can remember about that time?

2. What other things stand out in your memory about being a teenager?

3. Who were the important people for you? Tell me about them. Parents, brothers, sisters, friends, teachers, those you were especially close to, those you admired, those you wanted to be like.

4. Did you attend church and youth groups?

5. Did you go to school? What was the meaning for you?

6. Did you work during these years?

7. Tell me of any hardships you experienced at this time.

8. Do you remember feeling that there wasn't enough food or necessities of life as a child or adolescent?

9. Do you remember feeling left alone, abandoned, not having enough love or care as a child or adolescent?

10. What were the pleasant things about your adolescence?

11. What was the most unpleasant thing about your adolescence?

12. All things considered, would you say you were happy or unhappy as a teenager?

13. Do you remember your first attraction to another person?

14. How did you feel about sexual activities and your own sexual identity?

FAMILY AND HOME

1. How did your parents get along?

2. How did other people in your home get along?

3. What was the atmosphere in your home?

4. Were you punished as a child? For what? Who did the punishing? Who was "boss"?

5. When you wanted something from your parents, how did you go about getting it?

6. What kind of person did your parents like the most? The least?

7. Who were you closest to in your family?

8. Who in your family were you most like? In what way?

ADULTHOOD

1. What place did religion play in your life?

2. Now I'd like to talk to you about your life as an adult, starting when you were in your 20s up to today. Tell me of the most important events that happened in your adulthood.

3. What was life like for you in your 20s and 30s?

4. What kind of person were you? What did you enjoy?

5. Tell me about your work. Did you enjoy your work? Did you earn an adequate living? Did you work hard during those years? Were you appreciated?

6. Did you form significant relationships with other people?

7. Did you marry?

    (yes)   What kind of person was your spouse?
    (no)   Why not?

8. Do you think marriages get better or worse over time? Were you married more than once?

9. On the whole, would you say you had a happy or unhappy marriage?

10. Was sexual intimacy important to you?

11. What were some of the main difficulties you encountered during your adult years?

    a. Did someone close to you die? Go away?

    b. Were you ever sick? Have an accident?

    c. Did you move often? Change jobs?

    d. Did you ever feel alone? Abandoned?

    e. Did you ever feel need?

SUMMARY

1. On the whole, what kind of life do you think you've had?

2. If everything were to be the same would you like to live your life over again?

3. If you were going to live your life over again, what would you change? Leave unchanged?

4. We've been talking about your life for quite some time now. Let's discuss your over-all feelings and ideas about your life. What would you say the main satisfactions in your life have been? Try for three. Why were they satisfying?

5. Everyone has had disappointments. What have been the main disappointments in your life?

6. What was the hardest thing you had to face in your life? Please describe it.

7. What was the happiest period of your life? What about it made it the happiest period? Why is your life less happy now?

8. What was the unhappiest period of your life? Why is your life more happy now?

9. What was the proudest moment in your life?

10. If you could stay the same age all your life, what age would you choose? Why?

11. How do you think you've made out in life? Better or worse than what you hoped for?

12. Let's talk a little about you as you are now. What are the best things about the age you are now?

13. What are the worst things about being the age you are now?

14. What are the most important things to you in your life today?

15. What do you hope will happen to you as you grow older?

16. What do you fear will happen to you as you grow older?

17. Have you enjoyed participating in this review of your life?

*Form copyrighted by Dr. B. Haight, College of Nursing, Medical University of South Carolina, Charleston, SC 29425-2404. Reprinted with permission.

NOTE: Derived from new questions and two unpublished dissertations:

Falk, J. (1969). The organization of remembered life experience of older people: Its relation to anticipated stress, to subsequent adaptation and to age. Unpublished Doctoral Dissertation, University of Chicago.

Gorney, J. (1968). Experiencing and age: Patterns of reminiscence among the elderly. Unpublished Doctoral Dissertation, University of Chicago.

APPENDIX
2

Hot Lines and National Resources

HOT LINES

The following list of organizations maintain (at the time of publication) hot lines and/or Web sites, as indicated. This list was chosen for relevancy to the care of dying patients, and is not comprehensive. Current phone numbers can be found in any library that has a directory of 800 numbers or a current edition of *Lesko's Info-Power* by Matthew Lesko*. Or the National Health Information Clearinghouse can give current phone numbers. Call 1-800-336-4797 or Directory Assistance at (area code) 555-1212.

A useful tool for health care professionals is the *Health Hotlines* booklet available through the National Library of Medicine. It is a compilation of organizations with toll-free telephone numbers. It is free. Most are also listed in DIRLINE, NLM's online directory of information services for those who have access to the Internet or library facilities.

Government

Health and Human Services—Social Security Administration: Information on survivor, disability, Medicare, or Social Security benefits

www.ssa.gov   1-800-772-1213

Health and Human Services—Health Care Financing Administration: Referral service for second surgical opinions

www.hcfa.gov

*Lesko, M. (1994). *Lesko's info-power* (2nd ed.). Detroit, MI: Visible Ink Press.

Health and Human Services—National Institutes of Health, National Cancer Institute: Cancer information and publications

www.nih.gov   1-800-4-CANCER

National Health Information Clearinghouse: For ordering publications on health and some referrals (e.g., for laser surgery experts)

1-800-336-4797

National Library of Medicine: Information and reference database searches, 1913 to 1970, including audiovisuals (Current searches should be done online through local library services and interlibrary loan programs)

www.nlm.nih.gov   1-888-346-3636

U.S. Department of Health and Human Services: Health information and referral service

1-800-336-4797

Private

American Cancer Society: Information, publications, referrals, support groups (local groups may offer equipment and other kinds of help)

www.cancer.org   1-800-ACS-2345

American Kidney Fund: Information, publications, financial assistance

www.americankidneyfund.org   1-800-638-8299

American Liver Foundation: Information and referrals

www.liverfoundation.org   1-800-223-0179

American SIDS Institute: Clinical research, educational offerings, and treatment facilities

www.sids.org   1-800-232-SIDS

Children's Hospice International: Referral network

www.chionline.org   1-800-242-4453

Eldercare Hotline: Referrals to local resources nationwide

www.eldercare.com   1-800-677-1116

Hospice Education Institute Hospicelink: Referral network

                                                     1-800-331-1620

Joseph and Rose Kennedy Institute of Ethics National Reference Center for Bioethics Literature: Online searches of database on bioethic research (free)

                                                     1-800-MED-ETHX

National AIDS Hot Line (funded by Center for Disease Control): AIDS information hot lines maintained in English, Spanish, and for the hearing impaired

www.ashastd.org   1-800-342-AIDS

National AIDS Information Clearinghouse: AIDS publications, posters, databases, and videos

                                                     1-800-458-5231

National Hospice Organization: Referral and information help line on hospices

www.nhpco.org   1-800-658-8898

National Sudden Infant Death Syndrome (SIDS) Foundation: Publications, information, and referrals

www.sidsalliance.org   1-800-221-SIDS

Suicide and Rape 24-Hour Emergency Services of the Humanistic Mental Health Foundation: Crisis hot line, residential treatment program, and financial assistance

NATIONAL RESOURCES

The national resource agencies and organizations listed here are clearing-houses or referral points to help an individual find the help needed. This list is not comprehensive, but is limited to some of those agencies with the ability to help dying people. Addresses are given, but often a phone call brings quicker results. A few numbers are provided here.

A first call to the National Health Information Center at 1-800-336-4797 should be made to get the current phone number of the agency or hot line needed. Or you can call directory assistance in the area of the agency at (area code) 555-1212.

Bureau of Health Professions
Health Resources and Services Administration
5600 Fisher's Lane, Room 8-05
Rockville, MD 20857
www.hrsa.dhhs.gov
1-301-443-3794

Services: Maintains the National Practitioner Data Bank, which contains information on all disciplinary actions and malpractice claims or actions against licensed health care practitioners.

Centers for Disease Control (CDC)
Information Resources Management Office
Mail Stop C-15
1600 Clifton Road, NE
Atlanta, GA
www.cdc.gov
1-800-311-3435
1-404-639-7600

Services: A voice information system with prerecorded messages on health issues, with the ability to transfer the caller to a public health professional for more information.

Medical Care Ombudsman Program
Bethesda, MD
www.mcman.com
1-301-652-1818

Services: Free assessment of treatment options from a volunteer panel of top doctors.

CDC National Prevention Information Network
www.cdcnpin.org
1-800-458-5231

Services: Free publications, posters, and videos about AIDS; a fact sheet, guidelines for the prevention of the spread of AIDS in school and at work; and The Surgeon General's report on AIDS. There are two databases for on-line search.

National Health Information Center
P.O. Box 1133
Washington, D.C. 20013
1-800-336-4797

Services: Publications and information resources on most health topics. Referral and current phone numbers of any of the National Institutes of Health and hot lines available. This number should be called first to check for current 800 numbers.

National Library of Medicine
8600 Rockville Pike
Bethesda, MD 20894
www.nlm.nih.gov
1-888-346-3656

Services: Interlibrary loan; access to MEDLARS (Medical Literature Analysis and Retrieval System), an on-line database search system. MEDLARS provides access to other databases, like AIDSLINE, TOXLINE, CHEMLINE, HEALTH, CANCERLIT, SIDLINE, and others. This is the world's largest research library, and regional libraries will provide reference services and access to the National Library of Medicine.

National Second Surgical Opinion Program
Health Care Financing Administration
330 Independence Ave., SW
Washington, D.C. 20013
1-800-638-6833

Services: Referral to physicians for second opinion, and pamphlets to help patients ask the right questions.

Public Information Division
National Institutes of Health (NIH)
Room 305
Bethesda, MD 20892
www.nih.gov

Services: Free catalog listing publications available from each of the Institutes, addresses and phone numbers.

Public Broadcasting System
Web site on issues related to dying
www.pbs.org/wnet/bid/

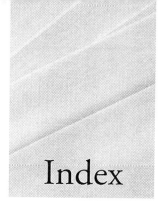

Index